I0767016

Vegan Doctor

Handbook of Natural Health and Healing

Dr. Philip Cargill

Copyright © 2019 by Dr.Philip Cargill.

All rights reserved.

Published by Dr. Philip Cargill

ISBN: 9781798073292

Imprint: Independently published

Formatted - Brenda Van Niekerk

brenda@triomarketers.com

Website Design - Brenda Van Niekerk

http://triomarketers.com

Contents

Chapter 1

What is in the food that you eat?

Eating properly

In your lifetime you may eat over 70,000 meals. Maybe a lot more. At least 60 or 70 tons of food. That's a lot of food. How much of it was good for you? What are your eating habits? What are the reasons for your eating habits? Most people seem to have an intuition about eating correctly, but just don't follow their intuitive guidance. If you don't eat a balanced nutritious diet, probably you will develop health problems.

One of the purposes of this book is to help you develop a good attitude towards eating. Good food and the right amount of it. I personally am a vegan for many years. I would like you to be a vegan also. It is better for the world and better for you. If you are not a vegan, you can still benefit from the nutritional knowledge in this book. And there are many other helpful concepts in this book besides nutrition.

I will be covering all the known ingredients in food. How much do you need? What is the purpose of the ingredient? I think everyone should know this stuff. When you eat. Think about what you are eating. What is in it? Where did it come from? Was an animal abused to provide it for you? Were farm laborers abused. Was the Earth abused? Eat with a clear conscience.

I remember reading about an experiment done with tiny tots. They were in a situation where they could choose their own food. Whatever they wanted and as much as they wanted. They were not given any other food except that which they chose. Guess what. They chose perfectly balanced nutritious diets. What happened between childhood and adulthood that we lost our ability to eat perfect diets. The more you know about nutrition, the better conscious choices you can make in choosing your food and especially the food for your children who depend on you.

Chronic diseases are those that are usually slow developing and take a long time to resolve. Many of these chronic diseases are attributable to poor diet. For some examples, heart disease, stroke, hypertension (high blood pressure), adult onset diabetes, and some forms of cancer. These account for 2/3 of all deaths in the US. Often these diseases are preventable.

Malnutrition refers to too little of a certain nutrient or too much of one. Either way can be detrimental to your ability to maintain good health. Too much or too little. How can you know? It is not possible to know exactly about your intake of food. Even with a super smartphone.

We all have certain indicators that we can try to be aware of. If you have a deficiency of a nutrient, there will be signs and symptoms that you can learn to know. Something is not right. You can sense it or it may be a lot worse than that. Pain or disability. And if you have too much of something, there will also be symptoms. The most common one for over consumption is weight gain. You could also feel toxic. Headaches, dizziness, lack of ambition and really, no interest in anything. Fatigue. Excuses for everything. If you have these, then maybe you have been overeating. Take a day or two off. There is no requirement by our bodies that we need food intake every day.

I am going to cover the basic components of food. Try to learn them. It will give a broader outlook on your food consumption. What is in the food and what happens to it when we eat it. It does not have to be complicated. I am going to give you a basic, simplified chemistry of food, and that is also the chemistry of our bodies. I'm sure you have heard the old saying, "you are what you eat."

Eating to attain and maintain good health naturally

1. Eat whole foods and chew thoroughly

2. Foods with natural colors contain necessary vitamins and minerals: reds, greens, yellows, oranges, blacks. browns, blues, purples and white is a color.

3. Avoid any food that is the result of the death or abuse of an animal

4. Eat fresh food whenever possible

5. Be very careful about the source of your drinking water.

6. Read all labels and avoid synthetic additives

7. If you have a choice, eat organic foods and non-GMO

8. Fiber in food keeps it moving through your digestive system. There is zero fiber in meat or dairy products.

9. Make sure the oils you ingest are natural. After opening the container, keep it refrigerated

10. Avoid hydrogenated fats or oils. They are synthetic.

11. You don't need any added salt or sugar

12. Eat a variety of foods. Many nutrients are complimentary to other nutrients in your food. Mix them up.

Those are some general principles for you to work with. You don't have to know every detail about every nutrient, but I think it is important for a person to have some understanding of the ingredients in their food. It is not just a matter of opening your mouth and filling it with good tasting food. Wouldn't it be better to know something about the food you are eating? Does your body require it? And why? There are not that many main ingredients for you to learn about. Basically, the same ingredients that are in your food are also what make up your body and keep you alive. Functioning. You can keep that information in the back of your mind forever. It will always be there to give you some understanding of what you are eating. Doesn't that make sense?

You have probably heard of all the nutrients somewhere. As you read on, the words and names will start to have some meaning to you. You might have a mental block against associating food with science. You can try to open your minds and even learn a little about food chemistry. This material is written on the level of beginning medical professionals to get some basic understanding. You can learn it also. Then you can read and converse intelligently about the ingredients in your food. Isn't that something you would like to learn? That knowledge can last you a lifetime and it will grow as you grow. Expand your mind about food. I would think it is something that everyone would like to learn.

The goal of proper eating is not just feeling full. The goal is the attainment of good health. Long prosperous life. Avoidance of being sick. Strength. Good habits for the rest of your life. Start right now. Start learning about what you eat and make wise choices that are designed to give you good health. It can be done. You can live a long life no matter about your family's health history was. It is never too late for you to start eating to maximize good health.

Carbohydrates

Carbohydrates are chemical structures obtained almost exclusively from plants, but two exceptions which do contain carbohydrates are the animal products milk and honey. Carbohydrates are made by a process called photosynthesis which takes place usually in a plant's leaves with a compound called chlorophyll.

I am not going to get complicated here, but basically what happens is the sun causes carbon dioxide and water to join and form the energy storing chemicals called carbohydrates. By the way, the by-product of this process is oxygen which goes into the air for us to breathe.

When we eat and digest carbohydrates, they are carried through our bloodstream to cells where they are used for fuel for whatever purpose that particular cell has. The name for the most common carbohydrate used for our fuel is glucose. It "burns" clean with oxygen. There is very little waste products except carbon dioxide which we breathe out and water which we use or excrete.

That energy was originally from the sun and was captured in the plant's chlorophyll. Isn't it an amazing system? The plant takes carbon dioxide, water, and sunshine to make the food and we eat it and get our energy and we give off carbon dioxide and water. It is a perfect plan. Plants and animals. Perfectly complimentary. Perfect because it was designed by God.

The plant makes the glucose into disaccharides or polysaccharides. As the name implies, disaccharides are a combination of two molecules. For instance, one glucose and one fructose, a related carbohydrate, forms common table sugar. One glucose and one galactose forms lactose which is the sugar found in milk. Long chains of glucose are polysaccharides. One example is glycogen which an animal stores up for emergency use in times of extreme stress. In humans it is stored in their liver and it is released during their "fight or flight" reaction during periods of danger and excitement.

Cellulose is a specially arranged glucose chain with complex branching that makes it indigestible to a human, although it can be digested by grazing animals upon a lot of chewing (chewing their cud). But anyway, Humans normally cannot digest cellulose and it forms fiber.

Food moves through the intestines with a process called peristalsis. When the fiber touches the inside walls of the intestines, it causes the intestine to contract and push the material along on its journey toward the rectum. If the food material has no or little fiber then the peristalsis is drastically slowed and that condition is called constipation. There is no fiber in meat or milk. Western man averages consumption of 2-5 grams of fiber per day. People in primitive cultures eat 18-20 grams of fiber per day. It is obvious which people are more likely to be constipated.

Fiber is often also called roughage and has benefits such as a feeling of fullness which helps in weight control, and as previously mentioned, it prevents constipation and hemorrhoids. It is also associated with reduced incidence of appendicitis, colon cancer, and diverticulitis, which are inflamed pouches formed in the colon. The fiber also binds with cholesterol and helps eliminate it with the feces, thereby benefitting the heart and arteries. The fiber sources especially effective with cholesterol control are oat bran, legumes, apples, and carrots. Wheat bran does not have quite as good of an effect on cholesterol, but it is a good stool softener.

When food is chewed thoroughly, there is an enzyme in the saliva called salivary amylase that breaks down many of the chains of carbohydrates. If the food is not chewed well, those chains pass eventually into the colon and are somewhat digested by bacteria there. This process causes the release of intestinal gas with the resulting flatulence.

Sugar

The world's favorite carbohydrate is sugar. Scientifically, it is called sucrose. We even have receptor taste buds on the tip of our tongues that react specifically with sugar. Humans love it. Kids like to lick it. Sugar gives us a good feeling. As I said previously, it is composed of one molecule of glucose and one molecule of fructose. It is broken down rapidly in the mouth and absorbed into our blood. A sugar "rush". Incidentally, there is only one food that the sugar goes into our blood faster than table sugar. That is watermelon. Everybody loves watermelon. I've never heard of anyone that doesn't.

Well, sugar is usually from natural sources. Sugar cane, sugar beets or corn glucose. So, if it is natural and we even have a taste bud for it, why not just eat a lot of it and be happy. Happy all the time. Back 60 or 70 years ago, Americans averaged 5 pounds of sugar a week. Now that we are more aware of sugar's dangers, we still average 2 pounds of sugar a week.

Too much sugar can possibly contribute to the development of diabetes and a lot of different destructive things can happen to us from that. Some people seem to be able to eat a lot of sugar and not develop diabetes. We are all different. Different metabolisms. Is there any danger to those people from excessive sugar consumption? Even if they are heavy activity people, mentally and physically. Both processes use a lot of glucose for energy. But there is still a problem.

Studies have shown that people who eat excessive sugar are less likely to consume what are called complex carbohydrates. You find those in real food. Yes, sugar is a food, but it is not adequate to provide for all the needs of our bodies. Complex carbohydrates have long chains of glucose molecules that digest slowly and provide us with a steady source of energy. Sugar gives us a big blast of energy and then we crash. The sugar blues.

Complex carbohydrates are usually associated with proteins, lipids, vitamins, and minerals. These are all things our bodies require for health and even basic survival. People who are resistant to diabetes should be able eat some sugar as long as they do eat enough of real foods also.

Bleached refined starch in white flour is almost as unhealthy as eating pure sugar. It is found in white bread, spaghetti, hamburger buns, cakes, cereals, crackers, and pizza crusts. The white flour won't hurt you directly, but it interferes in you eating food with more nutrients. The same effect is from eating white rice instead of brown rice and white flour tortillas instead of corn.

Here are 5 reasons that the American diet is so high in sugar.

1. Ignorance - we don't read the labels

2. Advertising - processed foods generate large profits

3. Habit-forming -sugar creates deficiencies and we crave

4. Convenience - junk foods are everywhere

5. Hidden- in a wide variety of popular foods

What happens to us when we eat a large dose of sugar? We become anti-social, angry, moody, irritable, and unable to concentrate. Kids become "problem children". We get withdrawal symptoms. Moodiness, headaches, fatigue, and cramps. The addiction begins in childhood and can continue through a person's entire life.

Sugar substitutes

Humans love sugar. Anything sweet. Most of us can easily get addicted, possibly for our entire lives, and our sugar addiction can add to obesity and diabetes, two conditions that can interfere with attainment of good health. There are many products that have been developed that can add a sweet taste to a drink or a food item instead of sugar, especially as a snack, or beverage, or dessert.

All of them have been tested and retested and further retested many times and there is no conclusive evidence that they are harmful to us. It is the job of the FDA to protect consumers from products that can be harmful. All of them have been approved. There are many people who fear any type of additive to our food and claim they are harmful to our health. Maybe they are, but there is no conclusive proof either way. So, if you want your sweet taste buds stimulated, you can eat naturally sweet food and let it go at that, or you can add sugar or a sugar substitute.

I am not going to go into the preparation technique of all of these sugar substitutes and no chemical derivatives. I am lumping most of them together as presumably safe to be used in moderation as sweeteners. Some may be better, some might be slightly dangerous. Nobody knows for sure. We do know that food is better if it is natural with no additives. Here is a list of the main sugar substitutes. I will do a little more detail about stevia because it seems to be natural from a South American plant, but for now, here is my list: aspartame, acesulfame - k, saccharin, sucralose, sorbitol, mannitol, xylitol, erythritol, yacon syrup, coconut sugar, honey, maple syrup, molasses, agave nectar, and corn syrup.

Stevia leaves have been used for thousands of years in Paraguay and Brazil as a sweetener in foods and sometimes chewed almost like a candy. It stimulates the sweet taste receptors on the tongue and also the bitter receptors resulting in a slightly bitter aftertaste, sort of like licorice. The coca-cola and pepsi cola companies had their chemists purify extracts from the plant that have no aftertaste and have been approved as food additives by the FDA just in the past few years.

It is from a natural source, the stevia plant, but of course, it has gone through considerable processing. It reacts in the mouth to taste receptors, but is not digested after it is swallowed so there are no calories. It eventually goes into the blood undigested and is excreted in a person's urine. It seems safe to use. Maybe it is the best of the sugar substitutes, at least at the present time.

Lipids

When we have excess glucose in our body we convert it into fat for storage. It has the same carbon , hydrogen, and oxygen atoms as glucose, but it is arranged differently and actually has more energy than regular glucose. Fat is composed of a carrier molecule called glycerol and 3 chains of fatty acids attached to it.

If all the carbon atoms are surrounded by hydrogen atoms, it is called saturated. Saturated oil is hard at room temperature like animal fat and butter. If there is one carbon not surrounded by hydrogen it is called monounsaturated and an example is olive oil. More than one carbon not surrounded by hydrogen is called polyunsaturated oil, like most of the cooking oils sold in stores and most of those are made with a lot of processing by heat and pressure.

It is much better if you can find a cold-pressed oil. It is more expensive, but what price is health. Extra Virgin olive oil is cold-pressed right from the olives and is considered very healthy. Other olive oils are second and third pressings after heating.

When we eat fats or oils, it goes into our intestines and is joined by particles of bile released from the liver that emulsifies the fat so it is easier to digest. Otherwise the fat is in large globules and it is hard for the enzymes that actually digest it to get to it. But with the bile the small particles of fat are converted to glycerol and fatty acids and drawn into the body. The fat goes into the lymph system and then into the blood. People who have lost their gall bladder which stores bile have difficulty digesting fats. Sometimes the bile can crystallize and form gall stones. I actually witnessed this myself. A patient had symptoms of gall stone blockage and recently his mother had died from a stone removal procedure. So he did not want to have surgery. He tried this and it worked. He drank only apple juice for a week. It has no fat and the bile built up a lot of pressure and then he drank a bottle of olive oil and the gall stones flushed out of the gall bladder and right into the toilet. He saved the stones and brought them to me.

Like everything else in our bodies, the fats (called triglycerides because of the three fatty acids attached to the glycerol) have a certain level in the blood and then will get stored in our fat tissue called adipose which is composed of a large number of fat cells mounted on sort of a netting. The fatty acids enter the adipose cells and the cells get larger. You don't make new fat cells, there is just an increase in size of the adipose cells, and really there is no limit to the size they can attain. If you burn off some of the triglycerides as energy, then the cells will shrink.

Since adipose is such an active tissue with the triglycerides coming in and out, there is a lot of blood vessels. Surgeries to remove adipose tissues often entails severe bleeding because of all the blood vessels. Once the adipose tissue is removed it can never grow back, but your body will store the triglycerides in other area, for example, in the buttocks instead of the belly.

Here are a few functions of fat besides energy storage. It carries dissolved compounds that give food an enticing aroma. Fat slows digestion, so we get a feeling of satiety. Fat gives us some insulation against the cold and cushions in some vital areas. Fats form the outer membrane of all the cells in the body. It forms an insulating layer around many of our nerve fibers. In fact, fat forms most of the white matter in the brain.

Like every other food component that we need, too much fat in our diet can cause us a lot of problems. Having a lot of excess fat means your heart has to work harder to be sure it all gets adequate circulation. How about the discomfort of trying to move smoothly when we are very overweight? Adipose tissue also has its own needs and add to your feelings of hunger. Yes, fat tissue calls for more nourishment, more fat. It can become quite demanding and can cause us a lot of discomfort with hunger. I will cover that later under leptin resistance and obesity.

Essential Fatty Acids (EFA's)

In nutrition, essential means our bodies cannot make it so it is essential that we eat it in our diet. Our bodies make most of what we need. Almost self-perpetuating. But there are essential fatty acids, linoleic acid and linolenic acid that must be eaten.

These are fairly important for you to maintain good health.

For one thing they make your muscles more contractile so you feel stronger. They work on the blood vessels to prevent hardening of the arteries and subsequent hypertension (high blood pressure) and also normalize your blood clotting functions. There are hormones called prostaglandins that are important when there is tissue injury and inflammation and those are dependent on the essential fatty acids, especially linoleic acid. Anyway, they are important. You have to make a special effort to make sure they are covered in your diet. Probably they are. You don't need a lot.

Linolenic is a type of Omega-3 fatty acid. If you eat fish, you are covered, especially tuna, herring, sardines, mackerel, trout, or salmon. They sell omega-3 supplements with DHA and EPA acids, but I personally don't like taking a supplement unless I was showing an obvious sign of a deficiency of omega 3. And even then, I doubt if I personally would take a supplement pill. Why not have a good meal with leafy vegetables, maybe some walnuts, some tofu, some canola oil, or especially some flaxseed oil. That's plenty.

Linoleic is Omega-6 fatty acid. Too bad the two names are so similar and makes it difficult to keep them straight. You need even less of this acid. Try eating some walnuts, amaranth, quinoa. You might have to make millet, wheat germ, soy. Also find it in lecithin and pumpkin seed oil.

Trans Fats

There are natural trans fats found in small amounts in meats and dairy products. They seem to digest well and are just another part of our dietary intake of lipids. What the big concern in health fields is the artificially made trans fats. Going back 50 years or more, there were large amounts of artificial trans fats consumed by Americans. That number has been steadily reduced as the American consumer has become aware of the dangers of eating it.

It has a long shelf life, so food manufacturers used it in a variety of products. It was considered safe. American kids ate tons of peanut butter that was not real peanut butter. Trans fats plus peanut flavoring, salt, and sugar. Now, most peanut butter does have some real peanuts in it. Margarine was a big deal. It was advertised as safer than butter and less fattening, and way cheaper. But it is made of trans fat and you certainly don't want to use an artificial fat for all the vital functions we use oils in our diet for.

For instance, the outer coats of all our cells in our bodies are made of fat. We should want those cell walls made with real, natural oils, not trans fats. You will function much better with natural oils. All our functions. Oils are important. They are in every part of our body. Especially in our brains. All the white matter in our brains are fibers coated with fat. You want natural oils for you and your kids. And before trans fats, there was very little incidence of heart attacks and cancer.

So, what are these trans fats? Industry took polyunsaturated vegetable oil, heated it very hot, lots of pressure, metallic catalysts, and they pumped in hydrogen gas, so it was now saturated fat but artificially saturated. It lasts for a long time without going rancid, so it gets used a lot in deep fryers in restaurants without going bad. But the food has the artificial fat on it and will be going into your body.

How about baked goods? Cakes? Especially if they use shortening made from trans fats. Also, cookies and crackers. Pie crusts. Rolls and donuts. Especially if they use ready-made frosting.

All kinds of snacks use trans fats. Potato and corn chips. Pretzels. Microwave popcorn. French fries. Canned biscuits. Cinnamon rolls. Pizza crusts, Dairy creamers.

Read the labels before you buy. Don't let your kids get poisoned with this stuff. The government allows the item to be labelled zero trans fats if it has .5 grams or less. Those .5 grams add up fast. Eat natural oils. They are very important. No trans fats. Nothing hydrogenated.

One of the effects of trans fats is it reduces the arteries' ability to expand. They become harder and work in conjunction with cholesterol to increase your risk of heart attack and stroke. They need to stretch if a clot is trying to get through a cholesterol narrowed passage. Eat natural foods. Not trans fats.

Proteins

We have glanced at carbohydrates and lipids. Those subjects could be dealt with in a full book each, and still not be comprehensively finished. Let's go on. You now have a basic introduction to those two classes of nutrients. The third group I want to discuss are the proteins.

Just for the heck of it, I am going to do a little of the basic chemistry of proteins. If it is really too much for you, then just skip it. I personally think it is important for understanding our diets.

You don't need to eat meat for protein. I'm going to show you why. Look at the muscles on cows and horses, and they never eat meat. As for brains, Einstein, Tesla, Freud, Gandhi, Mark Twain, Leonardo Da Vinci among many others got all their protein from plants and their brains seemed well-developed. I wish I had some of that. Let me try to explain how it works.

Basically, most proteins are composed of the same elements as carbs and fats. Carbon, hydrogen, oxygen, and the proteins also have nitrogen. These are all early elements in the creation of the Earth and of life. Nothing fancy. Life uses simple elements. I have to go back to our chemistry lesson briefly to try to help you understand a few things about proteins.

The thing about nitrogen, it is found in nature in our atmosphere in the form of two atoms of nitrogen held together in a very strong triple bond between them. Carbon, hydrogen, and oxygen are all found in nature with two atoms held together by single and double bonds and nitrogen has triple bonds. That means it is difficult to break the nitrogen atoms apart and use them in making a chemical structure, such as a protein.

Scientists use massive amounts of heat and pressure to try and break that triple bond in laboratories and usually they are unsuccessful. A naturally occurring enzyme called nitrogenase breaks the triple bond in an instant and the nitrogen will be attached to a new structure and it may be a protein. The nitrogenase is found in bacteria attached to the roots of plants such as alfalfa, clover, grasses, and beans. The animals eat the plants and are able to assimilate the nitrogen into proteins and DNA so they can live. Proteins are for structure. They can also be used for energy by the animal, but mainly they are used to form all the structures.

Proteins are made of amino acids. There are a lot of them in nature, including many we don't even know about yet. There are 20 that we do know that we use in our bodies to make our proteins. Nine of these amino acids must be ingested in our food, so they are called essential amino acids.

The non-essential amino acids are made inside our cells. Somewhere in every living cell is a nucleus that contains chromosomes composed of DNA. I'm not going to go into the entire process of the DNA making the proteins, but take my word for it, and read about it someday. It is an amazing process. Life is amazing to me. Every little detail. All the processes and chemicals that are interdependent and necessary for something to be alive, especially a human.

All the different types of cells in the body make their own type of protein. All cells are specialized that way. Cells are factories. Making something. Usually a protein. The DNA is encoded for putting the right amino acids together in the perfect sequence. Has to be perfect. One mistake and the protein will not function. We require perfection to stay alive.

Amino acids are joined together in a process called dehydration, a molecule of water is released when the two amino acids are joined together. The opposite reaction is called hydrolysis. It occurs in our stomachs. We don't want to use any other organism's proteins. We just want to use our own. And we are quite individualized that way.

We eat proteins from another organism, plant or animal and in our stomachs, we have pepsin which is an enzyme that make hydrolysis happen between chains of amino acids that we eat. We don't damage the amino acids because we want to reuse them. We just put water in between the individual amino acids and it breaks them apart from each other.

Single amino acids will get absorbed through the walls of our intestines and they go into our blood and lymph system and are carried throughout our bodies to the cells where they will be used to make our own proteins.

Proteins that we make include those used for our growth and maintenance. We build new tissue and replace worn out cells. We also use proteins to make enzymes which are catalysts to make chemical reactions happen faster and stronger. We use proteins to make some of our hormones which are messengers sent through the blood to make things happen. Also, we use proteins to make antibodies which are our germ fighters if somehow something gets inside our bodies. At last resort we use proteins for fuel. In the liver the amino acid is stripped of its nitrogen to make urea for kidney excretion and the rest is made into glucose for our energy or fat. The liver is just an amazing organ. It has so many functions to keep us alive.

Cells are sent messages to make a certain protein and that message causes activity in the nucleus and the DNA starts to form the long chains of amino acids.

Then there is a code where the DNA ends the chain formation and starts another chain. Maybe thousands of the chains in one cell. In order for the chains to be made all the amino acids must be present at the same time or the chain is not made. That's where you come in. Eating the right foods so all the different essential amino acids are available at the same time.

There is no vegetable food that has all the necessary amino acids available in prefect ratios for protein production in a human. Meat has all of the amino acids necessary for us to function. So does milk. Eggs especially. They have the highest form of protein for us to use. The best ratio of all the necessary amino acids is in eggs.

So what about plants? They all have amino acids, of course, but none have the perfect ratio of the amino acids for long term protein production. There are many people in this world who eat a lot of rice. It is a good food, especially brown rice, but it is not a complete food. They can't live a long healthy life by just eating rice. There is no plant food that is a complete protein. Eat something with the rice. Doesn't have to be at every meal, but a rice diet requires another food as a supplement.

You have to eat a variety of plants and then you will be covered. Different plant foods are stronger or weaker in the quantities of certain amino acids. Food combining is eating the foods that complement each other and make the perfect proteins. For instance, corn and beans. You're covered.

What happens if you eat too many proteins which becomes too many amino acids. They are taken in the blood to the liver where they are broken down. The nitrogen in the amino acid is used to form urea which is excreted by your kidneys and the rest of the amino acid is made into glucose to be used for energy or stored as fatty acid. Yes, you can gain fat from eating too much protein. Diet and health are always about a balance.

How much protein should you eat in a day? Some studies suggest we need about a gram of protein for each kilogram of our body weight. That figure is only useful if you know the approximate percentage of protein in the food you are eating. Then you figure out the grams of protein present in your food. Those figures are available on the internet. Some rough estimated values for protein content by weight are ground beef 25%, beans 10%, cheese 20%, eggs 10%, cow's milk 4%.

More protein information

Let's say you are 150 pounds. A safe amount of protein for you to eat in a day is a couple of ounces. Now that is a couple of ounces of actual protein, not the weight of the food that contains the protein. If you want that figure you have to see what percentage of certain foods is protein, and you can work from there. For example, soybean flour is 40% protein so you need 2 ounces divided by .40 which means you could get your necessary protein for a day eating 5 ounces of soy flour.

Cheese is about 25% protein, nuts 30%, meat 25% on average, beans 25%, grains and brown rice are 10%, eggs 10% and whole milk is 5% protein. There are charts on the internet, you can sort of find the protein content of most any food.

We are especially interested in the essential amino acids in our protein consumption. They are the ones we must eat because our own bodies do not manufacture them, and they have to be eaten in kind of a proper ratio at about the same time, or else some of our own protein synthesis will not take place or fall to a very low level. The biological value of a protein food is how closely it matches that which the body can use. In other words, the proportion of protein that can be absorbed by the digestive tract and retained by the body.

The term covering the protein digestibility and use by the body is NPU, net protein utilization. Egg protein closely matches the human body's requirements for Essential Amino Acids and its NPU is 94. That is the highest of all foods. Cheese is 70, peanuts are 40, milk is 85, fish 80, brown rice 70, meat 65, soybeans 65, nuts, beans and grains are 50. So those are measures of high-quality protein for use in our bodies. The first set of numbers were the amount of protein by percentage in food and these numbers relate the quality of those proteins for human use.

A person can avoid eating animal protein sources if they eat a variety of plant proteins which have complimentary amino acid patterns. All plants are deficient in certain amino acids. The idea is to eat plants that supplement the amino acids that are deficient in another plant food. For example, eating brown rice and beans together can increase the actual usable protein for your body. And the increase is substantial. Enough to keep you strong and healthy. ¾ cup of beans and 2 cups of brown rice is equal to protein in a 10 ounce steak, if the beans and rice are eaten together. Another example is corn and beans. ½ cup of beans eaten with 2 cups of corn meal is equal to a 5 ounce steak in protein.

Another consideration is the amount of calories you will ingest in eating the protein. To get 1 gram of protein from an egg you take in 14 calories. cottage cheese, 10 calories, whole milk 23 calories (fats have a lot of calories), cheddar cheese, 23, sprouts 12, mushrooms 14, broccoli 16, potatoes 60, corn 37, beans 40, brown rice 69, nuts, 60, hamburger 15, chicken 7.

Let's consider the approximate cost for our 150 pound person to get their 60 grams of required protein in their food. Prices vary a lot so I am just giving a rough estimate. You probably know more about it than I do. So you can sort of figure it out also. Whole eggs,$.20, cheese $1.50, milk, $1.00, cottage cheese, $1.20, soybeans $.30, most beans, $.50, Brown rice $.70, packaged cereal, $5.00, tuna, $1.20, shrimp $7.00, nuts $.3.00, hamburger, $1.50, steak $5.00, chicken $.70.

DNA, vitamins, and minerals that we eat

What about all the DNA that we eat? If you eat something that was alive then there will be DNA. Every cell that is from any living thing has a nucleus and there is DNA inside every nucleus. Sort of a lot of it. Well, it gets broken down in our digestive processing going on after we eat it. We don't use any other organism's DNA inside our body, so we just break it down into basic chemical components which we absorb and can use as we make our own DNA. And we make a lot of it as our cells divide and reproduce. It is one of the processes of life.

Vitamins and minerals? They get absorbed in the digestive system as they are needed. If you don't need them, then they move into the colon and probably will get eliminated with the feces. We need vitamins and minerals for many of our life functions, but you might already have more than you need so the natural vitamins and minerals in your food might not get absorbed. That is the problem with taking vitamin pills, especially multi-vitamins and minerals. Your blood becomes saturated with them and will not draw the natural vitamins and minerals from your food that you are digesting.

There are many people who would rather load up on synthetic vitamins because they don't trust that their diet will provide them with what they need. That whole attitude can go on and on. Take pills for protein. Take oils for lipids. Take carbs for carbs. Who needs real food?

Well, I do for one. I don't take any pills or any kind of supplements. I feel that everything that I need is in my natural food. If I restrict my diet to natural food, then I believe my digestive system will absorb everything that my body needs. Plus, I believe natural vitamins function better than synthetics. I don't believe that our food scientists can make a synthetic vitamin that works as efficiently as a natural vitamin.

How do I feel about a person stopping a long-term use of vitamin pills? How about easing off of them? Everyday take a smaller dose. By two or three weeks, you should be taking no more vitamin and mineral pills. You will be relying on your intake of food. Like real food. That's all. Nothing else. Chew it well. Eat slowly and when you are relaxed. No stress while eating. And no stimulants while eating. Like caffeine. And most important, eat natural foods. A variety of shapes, flavors, colors. No food contains all our needs. The key is a variety of food. Every day.

Water

Our bodies are composed of about 60% water. That's a lot. And we lose a lot everyday through our skin, through breathing, through excretion from the kidneys and also with feces. We have to replace what we lose or we become dehydrated. A part of our brain called the hypothalamus is responsible for our water balance. It measures the water in our blood and can signal the kidneys to not release so much water and also causes us to feel thirsty, so we drink more.

Here are some important uses of water in our bodies. It is the medium for our traffic of nutrients and waste products. Because water is incompressible, it acts as a lubricant and cushion for the joints and around the spinal cord and brain, the eyeballs, and amnionic fluid around an unborn infant. Water also helps maintain the body temperature.

What about a source of water for us to drink? There are not many places where the water is safe to drink untreated. Even the deepest springs now are often contaminated. What about tap water? The EPA requirements are often that drinking the tap water is palatable which means it will not make us immediately sick, but what about in the long term? What about the chemicals used to kill pathogens in the water? Sometimes they are removed by further treatment. Sometimes not. Tap water is certainly clean enough for washing, but maybe not for drinking or cooking. What about the many types of tap water filters? Using one has to be an improvement over drinking straight tap water. For me to say any more than that I would have to read a scientific study of the water quality after home filtering. You're on your own on that because I have not seen any studies.

There are three main types of bottled water available, spring water, purified, and distilled. Spring water is the least processed and contains more natural minerals such as calcium and magnesium. It does go through some purification processes and its quality is controlled by the FDA and the large food companies that produce it. Purified water goes through some sophisticated cleansing and it is probably the safest water, but not necessarily the healthiest. The natural minerals are mostly removed, but one element that is not removed usually is chlorine.

Chlorine kills most bacteria including our beneficial probiotic bacteria in our colon. Those help keep a normal balance in our colon and restrict some pathogens such as e.coli and candida yeasts. I read a study once that associated chlorine with colon cancer. Anyway, I don't like chlorines in my drinking water.

Distilled water is boiled and recovered and all minerals are removed. It is the purest of all the waters, but supposedly distilled water has a tendency to leach out our natural minerals from our bones because there are no minerals in the distilled water itself. Minerals have a natural tendency for equilibrium in the blood and any new water. So it draws the minerals from our bones if we drink distilled water. It is good for appliances that need pure water, but maybe not so good as our drinking water source. I have seen distilled water that has natural minerals added back to it. That sounds like a good idea. Probably a little expensive, but maybe worth it if you can afford it.

There are also problems with the plastic bottles. They have chemicals that can possibly leach into the water. One type is sort of a chemical estrogen that might have a feminizing effect on male users and cause reproductive problems with females. Even possibly cancer. And of course, disposing of the bottles is difficult. They should be recycled and hopefully not end up in our landfills or the oceans.

There are a lot of waters out there for sale. They each have some claim to fame. I have not tried most of them, so I am not going to make any recommendation. Here are large variances in prices. You are on your own. What your tastes are, what your needs are, what your price range is. Try them all. Study them. Pick out the one you like best and stick with it. You should vary your brand though. Like anything you are putting in your body, it is better to use a variety. No use exposing your body to the same things over and over indefinitely. And that goes for all kinds of foods and brands. Variety is the way to go. And safer.

Minerals

Yes, we need minerals to stay alive. They are important parts of many of our structures, and also necessary parts of the chemical reactions going on all the time. That is what makes us alive.

We try to conserve our minerals and reuse them, but some are naturally lost so we replenish them by eating whole foods. You don't need a pill or any kind of mineral supplement. You just need to eat a variety of natural foods. Everything has minerals in it or it would not have been alive. And I mean plants.

Chew it up good. It makes it easier to digest. The minerals are mixed in with our partially digested food and it sloshes against the intestinal walls. The walls are thin. Maybe one cell thick.

On the inside of those walls are little blood vessels, capillaries. They are also just one cell thick. If the blood has a shortage of a mineral, that mineral will naturally cross from the food into the capillaries.

It all depends on the balance. That is the way minerals work. They maintain an equilibrium somehow and the minerals are naturally drawn in if they are needed. If we don't need them, they go out with the feces. I personally think that is amazing. It just happens because it happens. The system evolved over a billion years. It works automatically. You need some calcium? Just draw it into your blood out of the food in your intestines. There is plenty. Just take what you need.

We also have storage spots for minerals. Like in the bones. If you are really short on your intake of certain minerals, your blood will draw them out of your bones to keep that equilibrium in your blood. We need the minerals to stay alive. Our bodies prefer natural minerals, not those high-potency synthetic supplements. If your blood is loaded up with those, then the natural minerals will not be absorbed. Eat good food.

I'm going to briefly mention some of the main minerals that we need. My mentor was the great naturopath of the last generation. Dr. Paavo Airola. I will draw on his personal research and knowledge as an introduction to our basic needs of minerals and the sources of them.

Calcium - we need it for our bones and teeth and is very important for heart action and muscle activity. Deficiency will result in things like osteoporosis, tooth decay, retarded growth, nervousness, mental depression, heart palpitations, muscle cramps, and irritability. Sources include milk and cheese, raw vegetables, especially dark leafy vegetables. Sesame seeds, oats, navy beans, millet, walnuts, sunflower seeds, peanuts. Too much calcium ca become toxic and possibly cause heart failure. Watch out for those pills.

Phosphorous - It works together with calcium for the strength of our bones and teeth and also our gums. It is an important part of our energy production from carbohydrates. We need it for our healthy nervous and mental activity. Deficiency results in weak bones, reduced sexual power, general weakness of the body, Sources include seeds, whole grains, nuts, legumes, egg yolks, dried fruits. Too much interferes with calcium, zinc, and magnesium absorption. A lot is found in soda pop.

Magnesium – it is a catalyst for many energy type reactions in the body. The reactions don't work without the magnesium. It just has to be there.

Strong muscles and bones. Helps in production of lecithin and will help reduce cholesterol buildup in arteries. Deficiency - kidney stones, kidney damage, atherosclerosis, heart attacks, seizures, irritability, depression, confusion, premature wrinkles. Sources – nuts, beans, green leafy vegetables, figs, apples, lemons, almonds, grains brown rice, seeds

Potassium – necessary for muscle contractions including the heart and proper functioning of the nervous system. Promotes the secretion of hormones. Prevents female disorders. Deficiency – Accumulation of salt in the tissues with sodium poisoning, edema, high blood pressure and heart failure, constipation, fatigue, low blood sugar. Sources – all vegetables, whole grains, seeds, nuts, potatoes especially with peelings, bananas

Sodium – many vital functions in the body. Become electrically charged ions which carry nerve impulses and is involved with maintaining the body's fluid levels. Deficiency -very rare because it is in so many foods. can cause nausea, weakness, exhaustion, apathy, respiratory failure. Too much sodium is common because of overuse of table salt and it leads to water retention, high blood pressure, stomach disorders, hardening of the arteries. Sources – kelp, celery, romaine, watermelon, asparagus

Chlorine – main function is to form hydrochloric acid in the stomach which is needed for proper protein digestion. Involved in maintaining fluid and electrolyte balance in the body. Deficiency _ impaired digestion, and imbalanced fluid levels. Sources - seaweed, kelp, watercress, avocado, chard, asparagus, pineapple, oats, sea salt

Sulfur – the beauty mineral. Vital for healthy hair, skin and nails. Deficiency – brittle nails and hair, skin disorders, eczema, rashes, blemishes Sources – radish, turnip, onions, celery, horseradish, string beans, watercress, kale, soybeans,

Iron – essential for the formation of hemoglobin which carries oxygen in the blood from the lungs to the cells of the body. Deficiency – nutritional anemia, lowered resistance to disease, run-down feeling, shortness of breath, headaches, pale complexion, low interest in sex. Sources – apricots, peaches, bananas, molasses, prunes, raisins, brewer's yeast, whole grains, turnip greens, beets, alfalfa, seeds, nuts, beans, kelp, egg yolks

Iodine – essential for the health of the thyroid gland and formation of thyroxin hormone from the thyroid which regulates the rate of metabolism and energy production. Prevents rough and wrinkled skin. Deficiency – enlargement of the thyroid gland called goiter and anemia, lethargy, obesity, slowed pulse, low blood pressure, lack of interest in sex. Sources – kelp, other seaweeds, turnip greens, artichoke, garlic, citrus, iodized salt, pineapple.

Zinc – involved in many hormone functions, especially reproductive hormones, involved in production of insulin and therefore, carbohydrate metabolism, normal growth of the sex organs and normal function of the prostate gland. Deficiency – retarded growth, underdeveloped sex organs, loss of fertility, white spots on fingernails, poor sense of taste and smell, hair loss, apathy towards learning. Sources – wheat bran, wheat germ, pumpkin seed, sunflower seeds, eggs, onions, herring, nuts, green leafy vegetables, sprouts.

Some of the other minerals that we need are copper, chromium, cobalt, fluorine, molybdenum, selenium, silicon, manganese, and lithium. They all our found in a normal diet and all of them can lead to symptoms if they are not eaten in your diet. You don't need much of any of these, but you do need some. There are also some trace minerals that are sometimes found in humans. We don't know what they do or if we really need them. They are toxic in large amounts, so it is better to just eat a normal diet to cover all the minerals and not take any mineral supplements unless it is proven you have a serious deficiency.

Vitamins

We hear so much about needing vitamins. Yes, they are necessary for humans to live. About a dozen different vitamins that we must consume to keep our systems running properly. But you don't need any mega supplements of vitamins. All of them are in our food and in a plentiful amount. You just need enough to get by. Most plants have vitamins because they need them also. So if we eat the plant we get their vitamins to be part of our lives. How about some whole foods? Natural foods. Eat the whole plant or at least, all of the edible portion. Chew it good. Digest it slowly. Eating it raw is best, but cooked is better than nothing.

Vitamins A, D, and E are fat-soluble and we store them easily. Vitamin C and all the B vitamins are water soluble and we have to be concerned about our intake of them. Not concerned enough to start popping pills. Just eat some whole natural foods and you will be fine. I am going to give a brief overview of the main vitamins we need and why we need them and where can we get them.

Different organisms use the vitamins for different purposes, but they all need vitamins. All life needs them. We evolved along with the vitamins. They changed as we changed. We really can't make enough of our own vitamins to survive. We have to eat some. And isn't it strange that the vitamins are in plants. Not really in meat. Our main sources are plants. We don't need to eat meat to get vitamins. It has been proven by millions of people every year that you don't really need to eat meat to stay alive.

Yes, the vitamins have a role in the plant. They are not just hanging around waiting to be eaten by a human or actually by anything. Vitamins are active chemical compounds and I believe the plants need vitamins to survive, just like we do. Does it have to be alive when we eat it? No, it can be cooked and still be nourishing with its vitamin content.

Vitamins often act as helpers in cellular reactions. Sometimes they are called co-factors. And yes, those co-factors are necessary. Vitamins can be protective to our cells. There are little chemical residues called free radicals produced in our natural reactions and those free radicals can be very destructive, possibly causing diseases and premature aging. Some vitamins called antioxidants can help absorb those free radicals.

The vitamins also are protective to the plants and also co-factors in their reactions. The more we learn about how life works and what is going on here and there, the more we should be amazed by the complexity. Life is one layer of amazement after another. Plants and animals and even microbes. Everything just works. Think about the millions of years it took for us to develop all these chemicals and their balance to keep everything alive.

Vitamin A - (retinol) builds resistance to many types of infections especially on mucus membranes such as in our mouths, nasal passages and sinuses, throats and bronchial tubes. It also prevents eye diseases and counteracts night blindness. Helps protect against the damaging effects of polluted air. Be careful with supplements because too much vitamin A is toxic. One of the especially beneficial active forms is beta carotene. It is actually a pigment adding yellow and orange color to vegetable, but in our bodies, it becomes vitamin A. Red, orange, and yellow colors make the food good for your lungs and vision. Deficiency – eye inflammations, poor vision, infections in respiratory tract, frequent colds, lack of appetite, scaly, dry skin, wrinkles, dull hair, ridged nails, poor sense of taste and smell. Sources – cantaloupe melons, red peppers, red grapefruit, squash, pumpkins, red cabbage, sweet potatoes, green leafy vegetables, butter, fish liver oils.

Vitamin B1 – (thiamine) helps make proteins, strong nervous system, heart muscle, aids digestion of carbohydrate and promote peristalsis, movement of food and wastes through the intestine, prevents premature aging Deficiency – loss of appetite, muscle weakness, slower heart beat, irritability, chronic constipation, depression, exhaustion. Deficiency can be caused by excess alcohol and refined sugars or processed food. Sources – brewer's yeast, wheat germ, whole grains, seeds, nuts, nut butters, beans, green leafy vegetables

Vitamin B2 – (riboflavin) essential for growth and general health, eyes, skin and hair, Deficiency – bloodshot eyes, sensitivity to light, sore burning tongue, premature wrinkles Sources – whole grains brewer's yeast, seeds, nuts, green leafy vegetables

Vitamin B3 – (niacin) proper circulation and nervous system, intestines, mental health Deficiency- coated tongue, canker sores, irritability, diarrhea, forgetfulness, insomnia, headaches, anemia, depression Sources – brewer's yeast, wheat germ, nuts, whole grains brown rice, green vegetables

Vitamin B6 – (pyridoxine) activates enzymes involved in fat and protein assimilation, involved in production of antibodies to protect against bacterial invasion, regulated the balance of sodium and potassium in vital body functions Deficiency – anemia, swelling, depression, skin disorders, nervousness, colon inflammation, insomnia, irritability, headaches, premature senility Sources – brewer's yeast, bananas, avocado, wheat germ, soybeans, walnuts, molasses, green leafy vegetables, pecans, raw foods

Vitamin B9 – (folic acid) works with B12 for formation of red blood cells, production of DNA for our genetics, skin and hair, healing infections, prevents diarrhea Deficiency – skin disorders, loss of hair, grayish skin, depression, fatigue, miscarriages, loss of male libido Sources – green leafy vegetables, beans, brewer's yeast, mushrooms, nuts, seeds, peanuts

Vitamin B12 – cobalamin) essential for production and regeneration of red blood cells, prevents anemia, Involved in many processes. Deficiency – pernicious anemia, poor appetite, poor growth in children, fatigue, loss of energy, stiffness, difficulty concentrating Sources – eggs, aged cheese, brewer's yeast, sunflower seeds, comfrey, kelp, wheat germ, pollen. To be absorbed in the GI tract there is a intrinsic factor required. People who don't have that factor must take the vitamin b12 in lozenge form under the tongue.

There are quite a few other vitamins in B family and they are all important for good health and functioning. If you eat whole grains, seeds, green leafy vegetables, and nuts you should have enough of those vitamins. biotin, inositol, choline, PABA, pantothenic acid, orotic acid, pangamic acid, nitrilosides. All the B vitamins are water soluble, so you really can't overdo them. The excess vitamins of the B family go out with the urine.

Vitamin C – (ascorbic acid) this is another water soluble vitamin. Excess vitamin C is excreted. Essential for the healthy condition of our cement between cells called collagen. It is involved in the function of all glands and organs, strengthens all connective tissues like ligaments and tendons, helps prevent infections like colds, protects against harmful effects from stress and environmental toxins. Deficiency – tooth decay, pyorrhea of the gums, deterioration of the joints, slow healing, premature aging, skin hemorrhages and bruising, varicosities, Sources – all fresh fruits and vegetables, especially rose hips and citrus, apples, persimmons, guavas, acerola cherries, tomatoes, turnip greens, green bell peppers.

Vitamin D – (ergosterol) necessary to assist the assimilation of calcium and other minerals in the digestive tract. Controls the parathyroid glands which regulate the calcium levels in the blood. There is a pre-vitamin D circulating in the blood and when the ski is exposed to sunlight, the pre-vitamin D becomes active vitamin D and when it reached the guts it promotes the absorption of calcium from your food. On light skinned people even 15 minutes a day of sunshine is adequate for the vitamin D production. Deficiency – tooth decay, pyorrhea of the gums, osteoporosis, osteomalacia, muscular weakness, lack of vigor, premature aging. Sources – sunshine on your skin, fish liver oils, egg yolks, butter, sprouts, sunflower seeds

Vitamin E – (tocopherol) oxygenates the tissues, reduces the need for oxygen, prevents sex hormones and fat soluble vitamins like A, D, and E from being destroyed by oxygen. Dilates blood vessels and improves circulation, healthy sex organs, menstrual disorders, retards aging, Deficiency – can contribute to strokes and heart attacks, loss of sexual potency, menstrual disorders and female sterility. Sources -, cold-pressed vegetable oils, especially soy and wheat germ, raw or sprouted seeds, nuts, whole grains, green leafy vegetables, eggs

Vitamin K – (meradione) important for production of prothrombin for normal blood clotting. Important for vitality and longevity, energy production Deficiency – hemorrhages, nose bleeds, lowered vitality, premature aging Sources-kelp, alfalfa, egg yolks, soybean oil, green leafy vegetables, made by bacteria in our colon.

Bioflavonoids –(rutin, hesperidin, citrin, quercitin) strengthens capillaries, protects Vitamin C from destruction by oxygen, enhances Vitamin C, prevents hemorrhoids, varicose veins, eczema, psoriasis. Deficiency – purple or blue spots on skin from bleeding, diminished Vitamin C activity. Sources – fresh fruits and vegetables, citrus, grapes, green peppers, apricots, cherries, prunes

There are other vitamins like F, T, and U and there are no doubt more that have not been discovered yet or named. They are in whole, natural fresh food. Eat well, and you will be fine.

Food safety

The greatest health risk from food is contamination by bacteria and to a lesser extent by viruses and fungi. There is also a smaller risk caused by food additives and chemical contamination.

Most cases of diarrhea in this country are caused by food-borne organisms. The cost is many billions of dollars a year in medical expenses and lost productivity. The illnesses also lead to thousands of deaths.

The elderly are especially susceptible because their poor eyesight and senses of smell and taste make it harder to detect spoiled food or dirty utensils. They also have weakened immune systems, low acid production in their stomachs to destroy the bacteria, and poor circulation which can prevent white blood cells and antibodies from reaching the infections.

Most generally healthy individuals who are exposed to food-borne microorganisms experience a brief though distressing episode of diarrhea, with no real long-term risks to their health. The following groups can be affected more seriously: children, the elderly, those with liver disease, diabetes, or AIDS, cancer patients, pregnant women, and people on immunosuppressant medications. Among these people, bouts of food-borne illness can be lengthy and lead to food allergies, seizures, blood poisoning from toxins, and other illnesses.

Often the contamination cannot be detected by taste, smell, or sight, and you might not even be aware of what food caused you the distress. That is why we must assume responsibility for safe handling of food, both for our own use and if we are preparing the food for others.

Here are rules from the World Health Organization: cook food thoroughly, store cooked foods carefully, reheat cooked foods thoroughly, avoid contact between raw and cooked food, wash hands often when cooking, keep all kitchen surfaces clean, protect food from insects and rodents and any other animals, and use pure water when cooking.

The current risk of food-borne illness is high mainly because of consumer mishandling and also because there is greater consumer interest in eating animal food raw or undercooked. Also, there are many people on medications that suppress their ability to combat the microbes and there are more older folks now.

Another factor is that the food industry tries to increase the shelf life as long as possible and that gives the bacteria more time to multiply. Cooked products are especially at risk even if refrigerated because the bacterial growth can flourish. And yes, if you are infected with a bacteria, the number of the bacteria is an important factor in assessing the severity of the infection.

The risk increases as more of our foods are prepared by centralized kitchens outsider the home. More people are looking for convenient east to prepare meals. Many supermarkets off entrees that can be served immediately or reheated. The meals are often prepared at a central kitchen and shipped to the store.

Even when the food is sealed in plastic bags does not stop the growth of many organisms which thrive on the moist nutritious contents of the bad. Even happens with salad sealed up in the bags. The growth of large-scale food production has introduced new and different risks than before. Another risk is from the greater consumption of ready to eat foods imported from other countries, examples are cheeses and seafoods. Raw oysters are especially in danger of being contaminated.

Here is a list of the most common microbial contaminants that affect Americans.

Staph aureus - found in nasal passages and on skin. Can contaminate meats, poultry, egg products, potato or macaroni or tuna salads. Cream-filled pastries. People think they have the flu, but it is food poisoning from the bacteria. Diarrhea 2-6 hours after eating. Lasts 24 hours. Did someone sneeze or cough on your food?

Salmonella – found in raw meat, poultry, eggs, fish. Diarrhea and cramps 6-72 hours after eating. Can last a month. Did someone touch your food after touching raw meat or poultry? Got to wash those hands.

Clostridium Botulism – found in canned green beans, mushrooms, spinach, olives, and beef. All canned. Neurotoxic symptoms such as double vision and inability to swallow. 12-36 hours after eating. Can be fatal. When you open a can, there should be air sucked into the can, nothing blowing out. That is a danger sign of contamination.

E. coli -Intestinal bacteria that gets into food from improper washing of hands or unclean meat processing. Intense diarrhea 12-24 hours after eating. Can be fatal. We have our own E. coli. The problem is if we eat someone else's E. coli and ours fights it and give off a powerful toxic against the invader. The further the invading culture is geographically from our own E. coli, the stronger is the attack. For instance, if you are eating in a foreign country, if you are exposed the attack will probably be stronger than if the exposure is from another American. Thorough cooking usually will kill E. coli unless the food is touched by unclean hands after the cooking. Use probiotics.

To avoid getting or giving diarrhea

When shopping, select perishables such as meat, poultry, and fish, last. Make sure they are put in a separate plastic bag. Promptly refrigerate or freeze when you are home.

Don't buy food from a container that is damaged or dented. Don't taste it if there is a foul odor or spurts liquid or gas when being opened.

After handling food, thoroughly was hands with hot, soapy water.

Make sure counters and cutting boards, plates and utensils are thoroughly cleansed and rinsed.

Frozen foods should not just sit unrefrigerated all day or all night

Avoid coughing or sneezing near food.

Wash fresh fruits and veggies under running water

Completely remove moldy portions of food. When in doubt, throw it out.

Use refrigerated ground meat in 1 or 2 days or frozen in 3 to 4 months. Ground meat is more likely to be contaminated than roasts or steaks because the bacteria has been mixed throughout the ground meat.

Cook food thoroughly.

Cook stuffing separately from poultry.

Once a food is cooked consume it right away or cool it down within 2 hours. Be careful not to contaminate cooked food with raw food.

Serve meat or poultry on a clean plate, not the same plate that had the raw product.

For picnic cooking, cook completely at the site.

Keep hot foods hot and cold foods, cold. Microbes thrive in moderate temperatures.

Reheat leftovers to at least 165 degrees which is hotter than

just normal eating temperature.

Keep your refrigerator below 40 degrees.

Be very careful about cross-contaminating between prepared foods.

If at a restaurant, watch for safe food handling techniques. Send back any food that does not appear to be thoroughly cooked.

Individuals who are collecting the money should not be serving food or handling food.

For microwaves, cover the food with glass if possible, to increase steam for heating the surface of the food. Stir or rotate the food and after it is finished, let the food stand for a few minutes to radiate the heat through the food

Chapter 2

Natural diets and weight control

Dr. Cargill's Vegan Diet

This diet is designed to maintain good health for a lifetime. All ages. Kids growing up. Pregnant and lactating women, Athletes. Intellectuals. Hard workers. Any walk of life. Older folks also. Guilt-free eating. Clean inside your digestive tract and your blood stream and clean spiritually. Promoting joy in life. Love for all life. No animal must suffer for your food or your benefit.

What about plants? I believe plants are on this Earth for our nourishment. They have their own life cycles. Animals and plants evolved together. Animals eating plants. Plants providing nourishment for the animals. Including humans. Everything we need to stay alive and flourish is found in plants. The plants draw the nutrients from the soil, and the sun, and the rain and then we eat the plants. And yes, often the plants will be killed, hopefully without any experience of suffering.

There are some fruitarians in this world who do not kill plants. It is a difficult lifestyle to provide for all your nutritional needs without killing plants. It can be done. There are many long-term fruitarians who seem quite healthy. I am not sure of the normalcy of their lifestyles. Spiritually, I would think they are on a higher plane than most everyone. I am sure they develop their regular eating habits just like the rest of us, except theirs is way more severe. But it can be done. I respect the people who do it. Actually, I believe that eventually humanity will evolve to the point where nothing is killed for food. Possibly all our food will be created by people and everything will be so perfect there will not even be defecation necessary. Eating will become of secondary importance. No more meals as such. Just a liquid or a capsule?

In this vegan diet, there will be some plants sacrificed to provide food for the humans. But as vegans are aware of the conservation of life, in a perfect world there will be no wasted plant life and the reproduction of the plant species will be preserved for the future of our eating. And the plant will be grown with a minimum of destruction or abuse of the Earth itself.

This diet is based on the word natural. We must seek out natural foods. Natural in the growing, the harvesting, and the preparation of the food. And of course, natural in the way we eat it. Stress-free meals. Eating slowly and chewing thoroughly. A minimum of cooking. Theoretically, no cooking. Eat it raw. None of the nutrients will be destroyed that way. The food is natural. From nature. From the Earth into our mouths.

No meat, of course, and no dairy products because of the abuse that takes place in the dairy industry. Dairy products do have a certain amount of nutritional value, but we don't really need them unless a person is going to starve without them. And that includes goat's and cow's milk. In a perfect world, people can get all their nourishment from plants. And we don't need eggs either, even though they are very nourishing. But we don't need them unless we are starving. This diet is based on a perfect vegan world. There is no vegan society at the moment, but every year there are millions more people adopting the vegan lifestyle and not using animal products for food or clothing or anything. Animals are for companionship, love, and enjoyment of their beauty and lives.

A key word for a successful vegan all-plant based diet is variety. Not necessarily total variety on a daily basis. If you have some good food available, go ahead and eat it. Even if you have eaten it everyday for a week. Go ahead and eat it. But not necessarily everyday forever. Maybe there is an impurity in the food. That is always a possibility. So take a break from eating it. And that goes for everything, including your activities. Try to avoid habits in eating and your lifestyle.

Color is important. If it wasn't then everything would be bland. Blanched. No brilliance like there is now in the world of plants. Colors are indicators that there is something causing the color and will probably be beneficial to you if you eat it. I like red-orange color for the beta-carotene to protect my lungs from the stuff floating around in our air. I like to start my day with a hand-squeezed glass of red grapefruit juice. Dark red. I love it.

Taste is important. You want to eat foods that stimulate your 4 types of taste sensors, sweet, bitter, sour, and salt. Not added salt. Just natural salt from the ground now in the food you are eating. We do need some salt to make hydrochloric acid for our stomach to activate enzymes that breakdown proteins. We don't need a lot of salt. We preserve the acid and reuse it, but we do need some salt for replacement of some of the acid. And the best is a natural iodized salt right from iodine containing soil or sea water. The iodine is taken from our blood by the thyroid gland and used to control the amount of energy we are using. If no iodine in your food, the thyroid swells up to try and look for iodine and it is called a goiter. If you cannot find food containing iodine, then you better eat some processed iodized salt if you are getting a goiter.

Bitter taste in food is indicative of alkaloids and those are good for us. Also eat naturally acidic foods with their sour taste. One of the best foods is lemons. And sweet foods are usually good for you. Naturally sweet. In our primitive early state of development, that is how we chose most of our food. If it is sweet, then eat it.

Mix your foods. Some of this and some of that. You don't need a lot of any kind of food. A little of this and a little of that. Different foods help each other get digested, absorbed, and utilized in the body. The nutrients work together. And I have a glass of natural vegetable juice with my meal so the nutrients in the juice can join in the party in my digestive tract. The idea is to get the nutrients into your blood so they can get taken around to wherever they are needed. Nutrients in one food help the nutrients in another food. Our meal is of foods that work together. Chew them well and mix them. They will bring life to your digestive tract and throughout your body.

So what about juices? Concentrated goodness. Fresh and home-made. A variety of juices and they can be mixed together. Different juices are complimentary to each other, just like variety in your salad or on your plate. Juices are not destructive to each other. You may also learn to crave the taste sensation of juices mixed together. Can you find green juices? Freshly made and full of green vitality. Diabetics should seek out juice from cucumbers and green beans and even make tea from the pods of the green beans. Maybe the most protection against the common cold is fresh carrot juice. What could be better to strengthen the mucus membranes of your throat, nasal passages, and bronchial tubes? Organic if possible. Everything should be organic if possible.

Raw, fresh, lots of color and white is a color, lots of real tastes, and mix it in your meal. No eating large amounts of one thing. In fact, no eating large amounts of anything. Why get stuffed and wish you hadn't? Small meals are better. Easier to eat and easier to digest. That is what this diet is all about. Easily digested nourishing food. You can do it.

And you don't need any animal products. Your health is better without them. There is nothing in meat that is not in plants. That is where the meat came from ultimately. From plants. The sun, the soil, and the rain. You don't need to eat the meat to get all the nutrients. Just eat the plants. I think that you can eat any plants and you will be healthy. And at any age or occupation. Just eat the plants. Eat the ones you like the best. You will be strong and full of vitality. No processed foods. They will make a mess of everything you have tried to accomplish by eating correctly. Natural foods. Keep them simple, plain, and natural.

In summary: eating to attain and maintain good health

1.   Eat whole foods and chew thoroughly

2.   Foods with natural colors contain necessary vitamins and minerals: reds, greens, yellows, oranges, blacks. browns, blues, purples and white is a color.

3.   Avoid any food that is the result of the death or abuse of an animal

4.   Eat fresh food whenever possible

5.   Be very careful about the source of your drinking water.

6.   Read all labels and avoid synthetic additives

7.   If you have a choice, eat organic foods and non-GMO

8.   Fiber in food keeps it moving through your digestive system. There is zero fiber in meat or dairy products.

9.   Make sure the oils you ingest are natural. After opening the container, keep it refrigerated

10.   Avoid hydrogenated fats or oils. They are synthetic.

11.   You don't need any added salt or sugar

12.   Eat a variety of foods. Many nutrients are complimentary to other nutrients in your food. Mix them up.

Those are some general principles for you to work with. You don't have to know every detail about every nutrient, but I think it is important for a person to have some understanding of the ingredients in their food. It is not just a matter of opening your mouth and filling it with good tasting food. Wouldn't it be better to know something about the food you are eating? Does your body require it? And why? There are not that many main ingredients for you to learn about. Basically, the same ingredients that are in your food are also what make up your body and keep you alive. Functioning. You can keep that information in the back of your mind forever. It will always be there to give you some understanding of what you are eating. Doesn't that make sense?

You have probably heard of all the nutrients somewhere. As you read on, the words and names will start to have some meaning to you. You might have a mental block against associating food with science. You can try to open your minds and even learn a little about food chemistry. This material is written on the level of beginning medical professionals to get some basic understanding. You can learn it also. Then you can read and converse intelligently about the ingredients in your food. Isn't that something you would like to learn? That knowledge can last you a lifetime and it will grow as you grow. Expand your mind about food. I would think it is something that everyone would like to learn.

The goal of proper eating is not feeling full. The goal is the attainment of good health. Long prosperous life. Avoidance of being sick. Strength. Good habits for the rest of your life. Start right now. Start learning about what you eat and make wise choices that are designed to give you good health. It can be done. You can live a long life no matter about your family's health history was. It is never too late for you to start eating to maximize good health. Sure, what you do with your time is also a factor, but first of all, the most important thing is what you eat.

The Airola Diet lacto-vegetarian

One of my favorite health writers from the last generation was Dr. Paavo Airola. He published quite a few books on a variety of subjects dealing with health. He was a naturopathic physician originally from Sweden and he also worked in Germany and also in the United States. He often referred to his Airola Diet as one of the most effective therapeutic ways to treat the majority of man's ills, correct diseases and restore, build and maintain health.

The Airola Diet is a lacto -vegetarian diet with an emphasis on these basic foods: seeds, grains and nuts, vegetables, and fruits, supplemented with milk and milk products, fermented lactic acid foods, cold-pressed vegetable oils, honey, brewer's yeast, and a long list of vitamin and mineral supplements. It is based on his lifetime of studies, research, personal and clinical experience and adapted to the modern age with its growing amounts of health-destroying environmental factors.

Fifty years ago, the majority of orthodox doctors generally dismissed nutrition as an important factor in health and disease. Nutrition was not even taught in most medical schools. Now most responsible nutritionists and many nutritionally and biologically oriented doctors agree that nutrition is a number one factor affecting a person's health.

Many outdated doctors and most dieticians believe that the so-called "Basic Four" food groups will ensure optimum nutrition. Many advocate a diet high in animal protein with lots of meat and recommend avoiding seeds and grains because they are considered food for birds. Some eat only raw foods, and some eat only cooked. Some eat only food that grows above the ground and some consider tomatoes and onions to be poisonous. There are as many beliefs in what is good for you as there are people who have opinions.

The Airola Diet is based on reliable scientific sources and evidence. These are the basic principles of nutrition for optimum health, youthful vitality, and long life.

1.   Seeds, nuts and grains should be eaten raw or sprouted but also may be cooked. They contain all the important nutrients essential for human growth, sustenance of health and prevention of disease. They contain the secret of life itself, the germ, the reproductive power that assures the perpetuation of the species. You should eat predominantly those that have been grown in your own area. The most wonderful health foods are millet, buckwheat, wheat, oats, barley, brown rice, sesame seeds, beans, and peas. Excellent sprouts can be made from wheat, mung beans, alfalfa seeds, and soy beans and sprouting increases their nutritional power tremendously. Complete proteins can be found in pumpkin seeds, almonds, peanuts, sesame seeds, buckwheat, and soybeans. These are also natural sources of essential saturated fatty acids, lecithin, B-complex vitamins, and vitamins C and A and E, which are the most important vitamins for the preservation of health and to prevent premature aging and many diseases especially of the digestive tract. Seeds and grains are also a goldmine of natural minerals for your body. Breads can be made with whole grains, seeds, and nuts. Especially beneficial is lactic acid containing sourdough bread made from rye.

2.   Vegetables. They are wonderful source of vitamins, minerals and enzymes. Proteins from potatoes with the skins, and green leafy vegetables, are of the highest quality. Food is your medicine and vegetables are your best medicinal foods. Most vegetables should be eaten raw in the form of raw salads. Some can be cooked, baked, or steamed. Generously use garlic, onions, and herbs and natural spices to improve y our health and turn dull vegetable dishes into gourmet food.

3.   Fruits . Like vegetables they are excellent sources of minerals, vitamins, and enzymes. Fruits are cleansing, easily digested and clean the blood and digestive tract. Use all available fruits in season and also dried fruits, unsulfured, organically grown raisins, prunes, apricots, and figs. Fruits are best eaten for breakfast and as snacks between meals.

4.   Eat mostly raw, living food. Numerous studies demonstrate the superiority of raw, living food for health maintenance. Many of the vitamins and enzymes are destroyed by cooking. Cooking also changes the structures of proteins and fatty acids and make them more difficult to digest. Eat lots of fermented lactic acid food such as homemade

sauerkraut and pickles. Sprouting is a good way to eat the seeds.

5.   Eat only natural foods. Your food should be whole, unprocessed, and unrefined. Preferably it should be organically grown in fertile soil and preferably in your own environment and eaten in season. Your health and longevity are in direct correlation to the naturalness of your food. Avoid denatured, refined, processed, man-made foods and canned foods.

6.   Eat only poison-free foods. Your food should be grown without chemical fertilizers and contain no residues of insecticides, additives and preservatives. Many of the poisons cannot be washed or peeled off. They penetrate the entire fruit or vegetable.

7.   Milk is certainly a disputed food. Some say it is excellent and others say it is bad and causes mucus and allergies. People who descended from countries where dairy cows were herded seem to be tolerant to milk and it can be of much value to them. The best way to take milk is in soured form such as yogurt, kefir, acidophilus, clabbered milk and homemade cottage cheese. These soured milks are easy to digest and also help to maintain a health intestinal flora and prevent intestinal putrefaction and constipation.

Goat's milk is better than cow's milk for humans. It also has factors for possibly fighting arthritis and even cancer.

8.   Cold-pressed vegetable oils. These are recommended as an addition to your diet if they are high-quality, fresh, cold-pressed, crude, and unrefined. 2 tbsp per day. They must be kept in the refrigerator after they are opened. Extra virgin olive oil from Italy or Spain, sesame oil and sunflower seed oil from health food stores.

9.   Honey. Natural, raw, unheated, unfiltered and unprocessed honey is the only sweetener used in this diet. 1 or 2 tbsp. per day. Has miraculous medicinal properties. Most centenarians in Russia and Bulgaria use honey liberally in their diets. Honey increases calcium retention, prevents anemia, beneficial in kidney and liver disorders, for colds, poor circulation, and complexion problems.

10.   Protective foods. Brewer's yeast, kelp, fresh wheat germ, fish liver oils in cold climates during dark winter months

11.   Avoid excess of protein. A high animal protein diet is definitely detrimental to health and may contribute to many of our most common diseases.

Proteins in excess of your actual need can be extremely harmful, especially an excess of cooked animal protein.

12.   Drink pure, natural water. Minerals in natural water is effectively absorbed and utilized by humans. They do not cause hardening of the arteries, kidney stones, or other diseases like arthritis and heart disease, even if the water is so heavily mineralized it is milky in appearance. It is becoming more difficult to obtain uncontaminated water. If you must drink distilled water add sea water to it, 2-3 tsp. per quart of the distilled water or add other minerals.

13.   Cleanse your system with periodic juice fasting. A periodic cleansing fast, perhaps once a year every spring for a couple of weeks can help improve our health, give our digestive tract a rest, and revitalize our glands and organs, and increase our lifespan. Juice fasting has been shown to be the safest and most effective way to restore health speed up the process of elimination of toxins and dead cells.

14.   Cultivate the following eating habits. Eat only when hungry. Eat slowly in a relaxed atmosphere. Eat several small meals instead of a few large meals. Do not eat too many foods at the same meal. Do not mix

raw fruits and raw vegetables at the same meal. Eat protein rich foods first. Practice undereating.

15.   Avoid the following. Tobacco, coffee, tea, cola, salt, alcohol, mustard, black pepper, refined white sugar and white flour, candy, factory made foods, rancid food, chemical drugs except in emergency, household toxic chemicals, and a sedentary life.

The Dr. Waerland Alkaline De-tox Diet

Over 100 years ago, Dr. Are Waerland and his wife, Ebba, ran a natural healing clinic in Sweden. Both had been sickly as children and they developed this detox diet that restored their health. The diet was so successful that eventually 40 clinics opened using this therapy in various parts of Europe.

This is the Waerland Alkaline detox diet

On waking: 1 -2 cups Excelsior Broth (see below) Head and neck self-massage, Cold shower, Dry skin brush, Morning Exercise or brisk walk

Breakfast: Home-made live yogurt & fresh fruit

Between meals: Herbal teas, Fresh fruit snack

Lunch: Kruska cereal (see below) with stewed fruit

Evening meal: Large salad including beets, carrots, onion, green salad vegetables, baked or boiled organic potatoes, plus sour dough rye bread, butter and home-made cottage cheese.

The program excludes salt, vinegar, pepper, mustard, strong spices, white flour, sugar, canned or processed foods, coffee, tea, alcohol, meat, fish, eggs and tobacco.

The Excelsior Broth neutralizes acid wastes, encourages the elimination of toxins and normalizes bowel elimination. It consists of a cup of vegetable broth with 1 tablespoon of flax seeds and 1 tablespoon of wheat bran added and left to soak in the refrigerator overnight. Next morning the drink is warmed to body temperature and drunk without chewing the seeds. The Excelsior broth is essentially potassium broth which is made from a variety of vegetables including organic potatoes with skins and water. No salt or stock is used. When the vegetables are cooked you strain off the liquid and you have your broth. You can save the vegetables to eat later if you like.

2 large potatoes unpeeled

8 oz carrots

8 oz beet (beetroot)

8 ox celery with leaves

Dark greens

1 onion chopped

Place all vegetables in large saucepan. Add 3 pints water or enough to cover vegetables, bring to boil, put on lid and simmer gently for 1 hour. Strain and drink only the broth. The broth can be stored in the fridge for up to 2 days.

Recipe for Waerland's Kruska Cereal

1 tbsp each or organic whole wheat, whole rye, whole oats, whole barley, whole millet grains

2 tbsp wheat bran

2 tbsp raisins

Coarsely grind the grains. Place in a pot with 1.5 cups water and add wheat bran and raisins.

Bring to boil and simmer for 5 – 10 minutes.

Wrap pot in blanket or newspaper and leave to stand for several hours.

Serve hot with home made or live organic yogurt or home made apple puree or other stewed fruit, with no sugar of course!

Waerland believed that the day should begin with a light breakfast that encouraged detox because the blood was most heavily loaded with toxins at that time. He said that a large breakfast interrupted elimination which goes on until noon so it is essential to have a easily digested breakfast which aided elimination.

Dr. Haigh's anti-uric acid diet

Presence of high uric acid in the bloodstream can cause gout. To prevent this condition, it is essential to watch your eating habits. Healthy eating could help you maintain uric acid at normal levels. Add the following foods in your diet.

Apples Add apples in your diet. As they are enriched with malic acid, they neutralize uric acid in the blood stream.

Apple cider vinegar Intake of apple cider vinegar is also beneficial. You can add 3 teaspoons of vinegar to 1 glass of water. You can have it 2-3 times every day.

French bean juice Drinking extracted juice of French beans twice a day is an effective home remedy to treat gout.

Water Water helps in flushing out toxins from the body including excess presence of uric acid. So, have at least 8-9 glasses of water every day.

Cherries As they have anti-inflammatory substance referred to as anthocyanins, it helps in reducing uric acid levels. They also prevent uric acid from crystallizing and getting deposited in the joints.

Berries Consume berries, especially strawberries and blueberries. Enriched with anti-inflammatory properties, **Fresh vegetable juices** Have carrot juice and add beetroot juice and cucumber juice in it.

Low fat dairy products Go for low fat milk and curd and prevent high uric acid in blood.

Lime Lime juice contains citric acid, a solvent of uric acid. Squeeze half a lime juice in a glass of water and have it every day.

Vitamin C rich foods These foods disintegrate uric acid and flushes it out of the body. Include foods such as kiwi, amla, guava, kiwi, oranges, lemon, tomato and other green leafy vegetables.

Olive oil Cook your foods with cold-pressed olive oil. This is a healthy start as it contains anti-oxidants and anti-inflammatory properties.

Celery seed One of the most popular home remedies to treat high uric acid levels is by consuming celery seeds.

Pinto beans Pinto beans are loaded with folic acid which helps in lowering uric acid naturally. You can also eat sunflower seeds and lentils.

High-fiber foods Adding foods that are high in dietary fiber absorb uric acid from the bloodstream. Dietary soluble fibers include oats, apples, oranges, broccoli, pears, strawberries, blueberries, cucumbers, celery, carrots and barley.

Bananas include bananas

in your diet

Green tea Consume green tea every day

Grains Eat grains that are more alkaline. You can consume sorghum and millet.

Avoid High-Purine Foods Including: Alcoholic beverages (all types) Some fish, seafood and shellfish, including anchovies, sardines, herring, mussels, codfish, scallops, trout and haddock. No red meats, such as beef, bacon, turkey, veal, venison and any organ meats like liver and kidneys.

Dr. Arnold Ehret's Mucusless Diet

Consists of all kinds of raw and coked fruits, starchless vegetables, cooked or raw, and green leaf vegetables. The diet also uses a combination of long and short fasts with progressively changing menus of non-mucus forming foods. Every disease, no matter what name it is known by medical Science is constipation. A clogging up of the entire pipe system of the human body.

Any special symptom is therefore merely a local constipation by more accumulated mucus at this particular place. Special places are the tongue, the stomach and all the intestinal tract. The average person has as much as ten pounds of uneliminated feces in the bowels continually, poisoning the bloodstream and the entire system.

Every sick person has a mucus-clogged system. The mucus is derived undigested and uneliminated unnatural food substances accumulated since childhood on. The mucusless diet was stated in Genesis, fruits and herbs and green leaves, but it has never come into general use. The average person does not understand what it means to cleanse the body of the quantities of waste he has accumulated in his lifetime.

Disease is an effort of the body to eliminate waste, mucus and toxins. For the body to be healed, it must be cleansed, freed from waste and foreign matter and mucus. It takes time. You have done wrong to your body all during your life. You need a housecleaning and regeneration and you will have clean and perfect health. The source of every disease, lowered vitality, imperfect health, lack of strength and endurance is in the colon, never perfectly emptied since your birth. Nobody on Earth today has an ideally clean body and no clean blood. What you consider to be normal health is actually a pathological condition. This waste can only be intelligently and thoroughly eliminated perfectly by the mucusless diet healing system.

The average normal man who is considered healthy has a chronic, stored up accumulation of waste food, poisons and drugs. Sometimes stored up for many years. These are latent diseases. When they are stirred up by a cold, he expels great quantities of mucus and feels unhappy instead of enjoying the cleansing process. If the quantity of loosened mucus shocks the system it is called influenza and sometimes can cause fever. Nature is endeavoring to save the human life and it can be called acute disease.

For ages the effort of nature has been misunderstood and suppressed with drugs and the continuance of eating despite the warning signs of pain and loss of appetite. Nature needs time to work and the patient's vitality and eliminating abilities are lowered by the drugs and the doctors will classify his condition as chronic.

MUCUSLESS: most fruit, fruit jellies with no additives, green leafy vegetables, starchless vegetables, sea vegetables, sprouts.

NON-MUCUS FORMING BAKED VEGETABLES: Acorn Squash, Asparagus, Broccoli, Brussel Sprouts, Butternut Squash Peppers, Spaghetti Squash, Sweet Potato, Zucchini

GREEN LEAF VEGETABLES (MUCUSLESS) : Arugula, Cabbage, Collard, Dandelion Leaf, Kale, Leafy Herbs (Parsley, Dill, Basil, Thyme), Lettuce, Mustard Greens, Spinach

MUCUSLESS RAW VEGETABLES/ROOT, STEM, FRUIT Celery, Cucumbers, Onions, Beets, Tomatoes, Peppers

BEANS (MODERATELY MUCUS-FORMING)

Beans (Black Beans, Black-eyed peas Kidney Beans, Lima Beans, Navy Beans, Pinto Beans, etc.; They are starchy, heavy, addictive, and mucus-forming,

NUTS AND SEEDS (MILDLY MUCUS-FORMING)

Nuts (Cashews, Almonds, Brazil Nuts, Peanuts, Pecans, Walnuts,

CEREALS (MODERATELY MUCUS-FORMING)

Well toasted 100% grain bread 100% wheat or quinoa pasta

OILS (FATTY AND MILDLY MUCUS FORMING)

Olive oil, Grapeseed oil

SEASONINGS (POTENTIALLY ACID-FORMING)

Onion powder, Garlic Powder, Dulse Flakes, Kelp Granules,

Oregano Granules, Thyme Granules, Basal Granules

VEGETARIAN/VEGAN PROCESSED FOODS (MODERATELY MUCUS FORMING OR POTENTIAL ACID-FORMING)

Chips (corn, plantain; Hummus, Soy Butter, Fruit Juices, Plant milks (soy milks, Plant-based butters (peanut and cashew, Texturized Vegetable Protein ('mock' meats including soy, etc.); Ehret discusses the use of protose–meat substitute made out of wheat gluten, Vegan Baked Goods, Veggie Patties, Canned Tomato Sauce, Vinegar Free Salad Dressing

MUCUS FORMING FOODS TO AVOID: Red meat, Milk, Cheese, Yogurt, Ice Cream, Butter, Eggs, Bread, Pasta, Cereal, Bananas, Cabbage, Potatoes, Corn and corn products, Soy products, Sweet desserts, Candy, Coffee, Tea, Soda, Alcohol

Macrobiotic Diet

The idea started around the turn of the 20th century. A Japanese army doctor, Sagen Ishizuka, noticed a decline in the health of the Japanese peasants who had adapted Western food habits. He devised a plan to get them back to eating their normal foods ad many lives were saved. One of the lives he saved was George Ohsawa who had been dying of tuberculosis. He worked with Dr. Ishizuka on his diet and he recovered.

Ohsawa had studied Chinese ancient cultures and systemized this eating system and related it to balancing the yin and yang of the food and also related it to Zen Buddhism and he called it the macrobiotic diet. His main principles were to eliminate animal-derived products, eat locally grown food, all eating should be in moderation, and balance the yin and yang of the meal.

Yin is expansive, light, cold and diffuse while yang is compact, dense, heavy, and hot. The foods he felt were closest to be in balance were brown rice, millet, barley, oats, quinoa, spelt, rye, and teff. The cookware must also be in balance. Use wood or glass. Avoid copper, plastic, non-stick coatings and don't use an electric oven. I would suppose that would also apply to a microwave oven.

Use whole grain cereals, legumes, vegetables, seaweed, mild seasonings, figs, nuts, seeds, fermented soy products, and fruits. By percentage of your diet well-chewed whole grains 40-60%, vegetables 25-30% beans and legumes 5%, miso soup 5%, sea vegetables 5%. Occasionally use nuts and nut butters, seasonings, sweeteners, and beverages.

Macrobiotics proponents do not recommend using nightshade plants such as tomatoes, peppers, potatoes, eggplants, also no spinach, beets, and avocados because they are all extremely yin. There may be a chemical solanine in nightshade plants that can cause a calcium imbalance and also lead to inflammation in the body and possibly osteoporosis.

Carb cycling

Sort of extreme regimentation of eating. At least I think so. I'm from the old days. Just eat what comes natural. Try to maintain a decent weight and rely on what seems normal and natural for you. That's the old way. Carb cyclers are kind of new. There is a lot more to it that weight control, but probably weight control is the driving force. But it doesn't have to be. Some people are just into doing everything for their health and body shaping to an extreme. To the max.

They can have a program on their smartphone to keep track of every bite. It can be done. And not just for carbs. All nutrients. You can get an instant reading about your diet, current and long-term. What you are missing. Maybe some things you are overdoing.

Most carb cyclers are following some sort of system of certain days with high carb consumption and also medium and low. As I said one of the defects is getting an accurate reading on your carb intake. You can get a rough estimate, but even that is unreliable. And you might bend the results to match up with your expectations and your food desires.

Another problem is guessing at your carb usage. We are all different. Some people can use a lot of carbs just sitting and doing nothing . Maybe their brain is being active and that uses a lot of carbs. Most carb cyclers adjust their carb intake to eat more carbs when they are more active, and eat less when they are in a period of less activity or even rest. That again is a generalization. We each have our own way we use carbs. Some people are more efficient physically and like I said, some burn more mentally when they are not being active.

I like the theory behind carb cycling and really, I believe all sorts of metabolic effects are possible. It is hard to do it scientifically though because of our individual difference and the many differences in the food we consume. Not all carbohydrates are equal. I really don't know how true carb cycling can be done, but I like the idea of it.

Ketone Diet

In our normal natural diet, the majority of our food calories should come from complex carbohydrates. They digest much slower than simple sugars and refined carbohydrates so they provide us with a steady supply of glucose that we burn for our energy. That is our normal way. The preferable diet for a human. Lots of complex carbs to make glucose. We absorb the glucose in our intestines and carry it around in our blood to be used in about every cell in our body.

It is possible that our blood has a shortage of glucose. If it is severe it is called hypoglycemia and can lead to pretty rough times including loss of consciousness and possibly even death. Maybe too much insulin released by the pancreas causing the sugar to be taken into the muscles or maybe a very restrictive dietary avoidance of carbohydrates.

Luckily we have an emergency source for energy and it involves the liver. First of all, the liver and muscles have a storage supply of glucose called glycogen. We use it in emergencies, such as danger and extreme exertion. Normally we store enough glycogen that we can function fine for about one day if we don't ingest any carbs. After that, we begin to draw upon our energy reserves stored in our fat tissue called adipose.

The fat is composed of two parts, glycerol which the liver makes into glucose and fatty acids that the liver makes into chemicals called ketones. The ketones can be used by the brain for energy. It is the only alternative when glucose levels are too low in the blood for proper brain functioning. In fact, the ketones work quite efficiently in the brain. About 100 years ago the ketogenic diet was used by doctors in epileptic patients and it worked. A least somewhat. Now the ketogenic diet is primarily used by people attempting to shed some of the extra weight they are carrying in their adipose tissue, their fat.

Does it work. For some people it really does. It is not easy. You have to keep track of about every bite you eat to avoid the consumption of carbohydrates. Is it dangerous? I think it is because it is so ab normal. I feel that this diet could be used safely in spurts. What is the big hurry? Take your time and alternate between ketogenic and normal food intake. How about a week of each? But that does not mean you should overeat ever. You worked hard for your weight loss. Keep it off.

So if you are not eating complex carbs or simple carbs, that means you will be getting most of your calories from proteins and fat. That sounds like a diet high in animal protein and associated fat. I am a vegan so eating that way is certainly not what I would approve of. There are high protein plant sources such as tofu and other soy products. I eat some of it almost every day and I really like it. It is not toxic. It is a very beneficial and healthful food.

I am not recommending the ketogenic diet. It does seem to work with many people however, scientists list many possible negative side effects from the diet. I am going to list some of them. Everyone is different, and the ketogenic diet can affect each of us differently. This possible symptom list is something you can watch for if you are trying the diet.

Diarrhea, nausea, constipation, vomiting, acid reflux, hair loss, kidney stones, muscle cramps or weakness, hypoglycemia, low blood platelet count, impaired concentration, moodiness, acidic urine, difficulty with minerals metabolism, osteoporosis, bruising, pneumonia, high cholesterol, atherosclerosis, heart arrythmia, menstrual irregularities, increased risk for heart disease, sepsis, mortality risk.

This does not mean you would be subject to any of these by doing the ketogenic diet, but they are a possibility and at least one scientific team is investigating it. Looking for a correlation. Just so you know there is the possibility of risk involved. Of course, being grossly overweight also has many risks involved. It is up to you to consider all aspects and choose what you will do or not do. Just so you know, there is no easy route with no risks involved. Think about it. See how you feel about it. The ketogenic diet maybe wonderful for you and it maybe destructive. Study it and you decide.

The idea to start the ketogenic process going is to eat high fat, moderate protein and low carbohydrates. We need some protein to repair our own body's proteins and build new cells and structures. You just don't need excess protein. It is better not to use protein for our fuel. It is not clean burning and has a lot of waste products for our kidneys to have to deal with.

If you are going ketogenic, you mainly want to burn fat for your fuel. Even in your brain. Ketones burn clean and will probably even make you feel better. What about vegans? Yes. How about coconut milk, olives, avocados, oils, tofu, nuts and seeds. There are lots of other foods also. High fat, moderate protein, low carb. It should work. You're on your own. I'm not pushing ketogenesis, but it seems to me that it might help burn away some excess fat that is really hard to get rid of any other way. Try it. Watch out for the danger signals listed above and if you get any of those, then I would say to stop it.

Women and weight

A recent study asked women "what would make you happiest?" 42% put weight loss at the top of their list. Success at work or school ranked top with 22%, a date wit the right man, 21%, hearing from an old friend, 15%. But weight loss was by far the most significant factor in their self-esteem.

The media promises women that with low weight and svelte figures, they will be happier in all aspects of their lives including improvement in their abilities. Obesity is considered intolerable. Even as children, chubby people are seen as lazy, less intelligent, dishonest, and sloppy.

A woman's attractiveness is tied to her ability to maintain a pre-pubescent body shape. It is essential for women to adopt other yardsticks for measuring self-worth and for improving it. Skills and knowledge must be valued and improved. And women must realize there are a wide variety of healthy shapes. And that must be backed up by appreciative men.

Men tend to attribute problems to external factors, women tend to blame themselves if something goes wrong. They blame themselves if their bodies do not measure u to the ideals presented by the media.

Many women feel that food and dieting is one part of their lives that they can gain complete control over and they may become obsessed with food ad the lack of it. These are prime candidates for developing an eating disorder.

A recent Gallup poll showed that only 17% of women eat what they want and that more than 80% dislike their bodies. Dieting is becoming a major concern in the lives of pre-adolescent girls to elderly woman. And the majority of women who exercise do it for weight loss, not for fitness.

Healthy eating habits lead to healthy consequences. They are thoughts and behaviors that are executed automatically in a response to a specific eating-related situation. Eat foods for nutritive and health value. Reduce the power of thinking about food. Feel safe to enjoy seeing and eating food. Know the difference between biological and psychological hunger. Respond to stress with behavior leading to healthy consequences.

Sometimes people attempt to suppress their natural appetite. Some feel hunger and physical emptiness is a pleasant sensation and satiety and fullness is extremely uncomfortable and must be avoided. Some people are functioning in a state of physical deprivation and are not living at a biological optimum level. Every human has a natural weight range which the body defends. If we try to suppress our weight below this optimum level, a number of physical and psychological symptoms may occur.

Impaired memory and concentration, loss of interest in previously enjoyed activities, anxiety and depression, mood swings, preoccupation with food, disruption of menstruation, constipation and other GI disorders, sleep disturbances, feeling cold, muscular weakness, brittle nails and thinning hair, and dehydration. Prolonged deprivation of food can lead to serious medical problems.

Eating Disorders: Anorexia nervosa

Excerpts from a letter written by one of my best students ever:

"I became ill with anorexia nervosa at around the age of 11. I had been teased as a child for being overweight. I am now 21. Before I became ill, I was 5'6" tall and weighed 145 pounds. I am now 5'7" tall and I weigh 85 pounds. My weight went as low as 80 pounds. Since the age of 13, I have been hospitalized over ten times for my eating disorder. Because I refused to eat, I spent much time being tube fed through a nasogastric tube.

I suffered many psychological and physical effects due to anorexia including depression, insomnia, emaciation, amenorrhea, fainting, dizziness, hair falling out, fatigue, and low stamina. Fortunate I haven't had any major heart problems, probably because I don't vomit or use laxatives.

Because I have childhood onset anorexia, I have a poorer prognosis. Also because 10 years have passed and my physicians believe I have very little chance of full recovery. The chance of dying from this are very real and frightening.

My body has adapted a starvation state because I've been sick for so long. I've been living on a diet of less than 1000 calories per day. My metabolism has slowed and I can live on this without any weight loss. I have huge goals for the future. I just may not be around to reach them. That's a fact. Anorexia will probably take a toll on my body if I don't improve soon. I will never give up fighting this disease. It has already gotten

in the way of me following my dreams. I will not let it get in the way anymore. My dreams are all I have left."

She died 5 months after graduating with honors from the University of Chicago.

Anorexia Nervosa - diagnostic criteria

1. For females – three consecutive periods missed. For males – impotence, loss of sex desire

2.   Refusal to maintain normal body weight

3.   Intensive fear of gaining weight

4.   Disturbed perception of body image

Typical characteristics -Rigid dieting causes dramatic weight loss, false body perception of being overweight, food rituals, rigid lifestyle controls, panic after a small weight gain, feelings of purity and power from self-denial, preoccupation with food, its preparation, watching others eat, helplessness in the presence of food, lack of menstruation

It may begin as a simple attempt to lose weight. A comment from a friend, parent or coach may be all that is needed. In an attempt to take control of their lives, may teens try to maintain extreme control over their bodies.

Once dieting begins, a person with anorexia does not stop. The result is a long period of rigidly self-imposed semi-starvation. The person refuses to eat enough. They are usually competitive, and obsessive. Often there is conflicts within the family, typically manifested by an overbearing mother or an emotionally absent father. Frustration with family expectations leads to fighting. There may be over involvement, overprotection, denial, and rigidity.

Often the eating disorder allows the person to maintain some control over an otherwise powerless existence. Losing weight may be their first independent success. Anorexics often evaluate self-worth almost entirely on self-control. Often they feel hopeless about relationships and isolated because of their dysfunctional families. They substitute the world of food eating and weight for the world of relationships.

People have actually joked about wanting a mild case of anorexia. Anorexia nervosa is not glamorous, but it has become associated with intelligence, upper class social life. Glamour, achievement, and perfection. Many patients actually pursued the symptoms as desirable because of these social connotations that have become associated with eating disorders. The disorders are thought of as afflictions of rich girls, but in actuality, the disorders affect all socio-economic groups, all ages, and men as well.

The pursuit of thinness never leads to lasting happiness. The more entrenched the eating disorder becomes, the less achievable is the goal of personal happiness. Quite often, the anorexic will die at an early age.

In general, people with anorexia lead depressing, restricted, and joyless lives, with feelings of personal inadequacy and overwhelming personal problems. Often, they are obsessed with food, socially isolated, and completely discontented with themselves.

Eating Disorders : Bulemia

Diagnostic criteria

1. Recurrent episodes of binge eating

2. Purging with laxatives, vomiting, diuretics, enemas

3. Binge at least twice a week for 3 months

4. Self-evaluation overly-influenced by body weight

Bulemics eat large amounts of food and after a binge, their self-esteem is low. Often they are perfectionists. Sexual addicts. Other compulsive behavior. Their teeth are eroded from the stomach acid from vomiting.

Their binge eating is secretive. They eat when depressed or under stress. The bingeing is followed by vomiting or laxatives. Shame and low self-esteem after a binge. Their weight fluctuates up or down 10 pounds. Loss of control of eating. Controlled life. Alcoholism, drugs or hypersexuality.

It is most common in young adults of college age. They are usually slightly above normal weight and they are sexually active. They know their behavior is abnormal and results in low self-esteem. Often they are depressed. Often they have been sexually abused. Inside they feel ashamed and frustrated.

Bulemics tend to come from disengaged families. Ones that are loosely organized. Very little protection offered by family members. Family roles are ill-defines with a great deal of conflict.

Bulemics often consume high carbohydrate foods during their binges because these foods can be purged quickly and comfortably. In a single binge 10,000 to 15,000 calories might be consumed. Even after purging much is still absorbed and weight gains do occur from the binges. After the binge the bulimic might feel guilty and depressed. Often hopeless. They gradually distance themselves from others and spend more time bingeing and purging.

Some bulemics believe they lose control because they are addicted to certain foods or because they are emotional eaters who turn to food in times of stress in order to feel better.

Actually, it is nutritional deprivation that is causing the bingeing. Negative moods or stress only triggers the binge for someone who is nutritionally deprived to begin with. The nutritional deprivation can be habit forming and can cause vicious cycles of bingeing and guilt. The prolonged effects of nutritional deprivation can be serious and lead to medical complications. With the normalization of eating habits, those symptoms may improve.

Healthy eating habits lead to healthy consequences. They are thoughts and behaviors that are executed automatically in a response to a specific eating-related situation. Eat foods for nutritive and health value. Reduce the power of thinking about food. Feel safe to enjoy seeing and eating food. Know the difference between biological and psychological hunger. Respond to stress with behavior leading to healthy consequences.

Sometimes people attempt to suppress their natural appetite. Some feel hunger and physical emptiness is a pleasant sensation and satiety and fullness is extremely uncomfortable and must be avoided. Some people are functioning in a state of physical deprivation and are not living at a biological optimum level. Every human has a natural weight range which the body defends. If we try to suppress our weight below this optimum level, a number of physical and psychological symptoms may occur.

Impaired memory and concentration, loss of interest in previously enjoyed activities, anxiety and depression, mood swings, preoccupation with food, disruption of menstruation, constipation and other GI disorders, sleep disturbances, feeling cold, muscular weakness, brittle nails and thinning hair, and dehydration. Prolonged deprivation of food can lead to serious medical problems.

Weight Control

1/4 of American men and nearly 1/2 of American women are concerned about weight control. 1/3 of American adults are considered obese and the number is growing. In the 50 to 70 age group 42% of men and 52% of women are obese.

Energy balance is energy intake minus energy expenditure. If intake is greater it is considered a positive balance the result will be weight gain. During childhood and when a woman is pregnant, a positive balance is necessary. Adulthood can be a time of creeping weight gain that eventually turns into obesity.

The body uses energy for three main purposes.

1. Basal metabolism – represents the minimal amount of energy to keep an awake, resting individual, alive. This usually amounts to 60 to 70% of the energy a person uses. About 1 calorie per kilogram of body weight per hour. 110 pound person is 55 kg so that is 1320 calories per day. The BMR declines as a person gets older and also if energy intake is low. Physical activity helps keep the BMR high so more calories are burned. More calcium in the diet also burns more calories.

2. Physical activity increases energy expenditure 25-40%. One of the main causes of obesity in the US is the lack of activity. The alternative to obesity is movement.

3. Thermic effect – we use energy to digest absorb and process our food. Almost 10% of our calories.

   We have two main drives that influence our desire to eat.

1. Hunger -controlled by the hypothalamus that is stimulated by the amount of glucose in the blood, also affected by other hormone levels, stress, mood, diseases, psychopathologies, and also by the amount of food in our stomach

2. Appetite – controlled by external factors such as temperature, humidity, social influences such as others present, and cultural traditions, odors, and taste, learned preferences such as sugar, salt, alcohol, and energy requirements.

Typical health problems associated with obesity: increased risk in surgery, diabetes, high blood pressure, heart disease, arthritis, gall stones, pregnancy risks, and premature death, various forms of cancer, sleep disorders, social discrimination so likely to have lower income, decreased chance of marriage, fewer choices in clothing, and rude remarks.

Body fat be measured by underwater weighing, skin flap measurements, bioelectric impedance and infrared light measurement. Testosterone encourages upper body fat storage, which is more dangerous as a risk factor for heart disease. Estrogen encourages low body fat storage which is harder to get rid of. Only a small portion of women have upper body obesity. Both genetic factors and psychological factors can increase the risk for obesity.

Sometimes individuals inherit a thrifty metabolism, one that uses energy frugally and enables them to store more fat. Families with lower metabolic rates have a tendency toward obesity. Also, certain ethnic groups such as native Americans. A child with no obese parents has only a 10% chance of becoming obese, one obese parent and the chance becomes 40% and two obese parents, the chance of that child being obese becomes 80%.

Poverty is also often associated with obesity, especially in women. Adult obesity in women is often linked to childhood obesity. In women periods of boredom or stress can lead to weight gain and the also pregnancy. Male obesity is often associated with sedentary lifestyle. We seem to have a natural level of weight that we try to maintain and when you consider the many tons of food we eat in our lifetime, our weight gain is really only a small amount.

Much of the mania concerning weight loss usually results from an unrealistic weight expectation, especially among women. The body defends itself against weight loss. During periods of low food intake, the body's metabolism is slowed.

Weight cycling is common with commercial weight loss programs. Only about 5% of people keep the weight off. One third of the weight is regained after one year of being off the program and almost all is regained within two years. Often the person ends of gaining even more weight than they lost. If the weight loss is lean mass then the metabolic rate will slow and further loss will be even more difficult. Weight loss and subsequent maintenance of that lower weight are possible, but takes extreme motivation.

Here are some suggestions: first reduce high fat foods, drink water before a meal, eat low calorie snacks especially before going out, shop for food after eating, use a shopping list, avoid ready to eat food, eat meals at regular times, women should gain no more than 10 or 15 pounds after age 21, store food out of sight, keep food off the table when not being eaten, use smaller dishes, avoid alcoholic beverages, practice polite ways to decline food, put the fork down between mouthfuls, chew thoroughly, do nothing else while eating, keep a diet diary, avoid unreasonable goals, think about your progress, plan specific rewards, pause in the middle of the meal, and only eat when you are hungry.

Leptin resistance and obesity

Leptin is a hormone messenger produced by our adipose fat cells. So the more fat you have, the more leptin is made and enters the bloodstream and is carried to a part of the brain called the hypothalamus which measures the amount of leptin and if it is high enough, it shuts off our feelings of hunger. We don't need to eat anymore. Satiety. It over-rules the signals from the ghrelin hormone made in the stomach that causes us to feel hunger.

A high leptin level also stimulates us to burn more energy. Even when we are resting. That is because the hypothalamus sends a signal to our pituitary gland that sends a signal to the thyroid gland to release more thyroid hormone which increases our metabolism throughout the body. We burn more energy and at least theoretically, we will lose some weight.

It is like a feedback system. Negative feedback. If there is a lot of leptin given off by our very plump fat cells, then we don't have hunger. That is natural. If leptin levels are lower because we don't have as much fat, then we do have hunger. Our brain thinks we are starving and puts some heavy pressure on us to find food and eat it. Right away. And a lot of it.

We get very hungry and it is difficult to fight off that feeling. That's why many people who lose weight on a diet, regain it again. We have less fat after the diet and less leptin is sent to the brain, and so our body craves food. If our leptin is low from less fat, we also conserve our energy by not releasing as much thyroid hormone and don't burn the fat. Just slow everything down. It is like our natural instinct to prevent starvation and deep instincts like that have a strong control on our minds.

Scientists suspect there is a condition called leptin resistance that could contribute to obesity. Even if you have an abundance of fat and you are producing a lot of leptin, if the hypothalamus wrongly interprets your high leptin levels as low, your brain is stimulated to go into the starvation mode, and we need more food and seek it and eat it and we also reduce our energy being burned. In other words, the fat should normally get used up for energy, but instead we eat more and gain more fat in our cells. Just the opposite of what high eptin levels usually accomplish. People can try to resist the brain's call for more food, but it is very difficult. It is also very difficult to lose weight if we are not burning a lot of energy.

So leptin resistance causes the hypothalamus to make a mistake in measuring the amount of leptin. Even though you have a lot of fat your brain is fooled into calling for more food. Nobody knows for sure what causes this leptin resistance. I think maybe the amount of leptin in the blood of obese people overwhelms the sensors in the hypothalamus and the feedback system shuts off.

Other scientists now think there is actually a disease process going on and the hypothalamus is impeded by being inflamed from the high leptin levels or from high amounts of triglycerides in the blood. Nobody knows for sure what causes the malfunction, and nobody knows for sure if there is a malfunction, but it a good explanation for increased obesity.

Does it do any good to eat foods containing the actual leptin hormone molecule. Or supplements with leptin powder or pills? It might help. It won't hurt to try it, although if you are obese you probably do not have a shortage of leptin in your blood. Probably you already have an excess and your hypothalamus is resistant to it. But it is worth trying. One problem is that leptin is a protein and will probably be digested into its component amino acids in your stomach, so I am skeptical as to the efficacy of the supplements or leptin containing food items. It is possible, though unlikely, that your fat tissue is not producing enough leptin.

Anyway, it is doubtful that any leptin can get past the stomach's digestive juices intact and still usable. It has to be made in the fat cells. Just eat natural, whole foods. Avoid processed food, extra fats, sugars, and salt. Eat good food and let nature cure you of any disturbance to your natural systems.

Planetary Health Diet

An international team of scientists has developed a diet to improve health while ensuring sustainable food production to reduce further damage to the planet. The "planetary health diet" is based on cutting red meat and sugar consumption in half and upping intake of fruits, vegetables and nuts. It can prevent millions of premature deaths without harming the planet. The report was published in the medical journal The Lancet.

3 billion people across the world are under and over nourished -- and food production is overstepping environmental targets, driving climate change,

biodiversity loss and pollution. The world's population is set to reach 10 billion people by 2050; that will worsen risks to people and the planet. Now 1 billion people live in hunger and 2 billion people eat too much of the wrong foods. Nutrition has failed to get the kind of political attention that is given to diseases such as AIDS, tuberculosis, and malaria.

This diet advises people to consume 2,500 calories per day, which is slightly more than what people are eating today. People should eat a "variety of plant-based foods, low amounts of animal-based foods, unsaturated rather than saturated fats, and few refined grains, highly processed foods and added sugars.

Some countries are not able to grow enough food because they could be lacking resilient crops, while in other countries, unhealthy foods are heavily promoted. There must be subsidies that move away from meat production, and environmental changes, such as limits on how much fertilizer can be used or we won't see people meeting this target. At the present time North Americans eat 6.5 times more red meat than is recommended and South Asians eat twice as much refined starches.

Prohibit land clearing and remove subsidies to world fisheries. Farmers must shift food production away from large quantities of a few crops to diverse production of nutritious crops.

Healthy food must be made more accessible to low-income people to avoid continued poor nutrition. Agriculture must take local conditions into account to ensure the best practices for a region and produce the best crops. Reduce food waste by improving harvest planning and market access in low and middle-income countries, while improving shopping habits of consumers in high-income countries.

Designing sustainable food systems that can deliver healthy diets for a growing and wealthier world population presents a formidable challenge. Nothing less than a new global agricultural revolution. It is about behavioral change. It's about technologies. It's about policies. It's about regulations. It can be done.

Eating to attain and maintain good health naturally

1.   Eat whole foods and chew thoroughly

2.   Foods with natural colors contain necessary vitamins and minerals: reds, greens, yellows,

oranges, blacks. browns, blues, purples and white is a color.

3.   Avoid any food that is the result of the death or abuse of an animal

4.   Eat fresh food whenever possible

5.   Be very careful about the source of your drinking water.

6.   Read all labels and avoid synthetic additives

7.   If you have a choice, eat organic foods and non-GMO

8.   Fiber in food keeps it moving through your digestive system. There is zero fiber in meat or dairy products.

9.   Make sure the oils you ingest are natural. After opening the container, keep it refrigerated

10. Avoid hydrogenated fats or oils. They are synthetic.

11. You don't need any added salt or sugar

12. Eat a variety of foods. Many nutrients are complimentary to other nutrients in your food. Mix them up.

Snacks

I asked some people what would be good snacks with no sugar, low calories, natural with nothing artificial, and preferably vegan

Rice cakes with different flavors

Celery.

Water

Carrots

Roasted organic seaweed

Oatmeal with dried berries refrigerated

Bananas and nuts

Salads

Sliced apples dipped in melted almond butter.

Sliced apples with peanut butter.

Natural peanut butter on seed bread

Baked sweet with chives and onions

Veggie lovers pizza

Nuts.

Walnuts

Smoked almonds

Bananas, Apples, Nuts, Carrots, Celery

Celery with natural peanut or almond butter

Dried plums

Guacamole

Broccoli, green apples, grapes, strawberries, blueberries.

Snap peas are good and sweet.

Cauliflower puffs

Simple Mills crackers

Apples sliced and sprinkled with cinnamon

Frozen pineapple

Organic snack mix

Granola bars

Sweet potato chips

Pecans, celery, cut up carrots, soy, pistachio, nuts.

Hard soup makers that you are supposed to add
    water to

Raisin

Sunflower seeds

Popcorn

fruit vegetables

Roasted pumpkin seeds

Boiled okra

Fugi Apple with smooth peanut butter

Dates, nuts, dried apricots, hummus and veggies.

Guacamole in a warm corn tortilla.

Fresh nuts in shell

Coconut chips

Dehydrated (freeze dried) fruit.

Pulp from juicer made into chips and crackers in
    oven

Celery

Energy balls

Dates and cashews

Inca corn

Strawberries

Celery Sticks with natural peanut butter.

Rice cakes. apple cinnamon flavored

Raw cauliflower

Fresh grapes

Nuts

Bananas

Wheat germ, sugarless peanut butter with honey

Edamame beans. I love them

Jane Peach Flambee Smith with nutritional yeast

Carrots celery tomatoes lettuce

Celery with fresh ground almond butter

Roasted chickpeas

Peanuts, cashews, pistachios or macadamias

A piece of fruit

Cashews

Peanut butter on celery topped with raisins

Some grocery stores allow U to make your own
    peanut butter

Soft Tofu blended with fruit

Roasted peanuts, or dried cranberries with
    walnuts.

Almonds and grapes

Dates, dried pineapple

Sliced apples dipped in peanut butter

Dates

Hummus chips

Unsalted almonds

Cucumber with peanut butter.

Popcorn from an air blower.

Raw almonds and dried apricots

Coconut

Homemade Oatmeal pancakes with peanut
butter and bananas

Chapter 3

Diseases, disorders, conditions

Achalasia

Achalasia is a serious condition that affects your esophagus. The lower esophageal sphincter (LES) is a muscular ring that closes off the esophagus from the stomach. If you have achalasia, your LES fails to open up during swallowing, which it's supposed to do. This leads to a backup of food within your esophagus.

The tight lower esophageal sphincter causes the part of the esophagus above it to enlarge greatly. This enlargement contributes to many of the symptoms. Difficulty swallowing (dysphagia) both solids and liquids is the main symptom. Although less common, chest pain may occur during swallowing or for no apparent reason. About one third of people who have achalasia spit up (regurgitate) undigested food. If spitting up occurs when people are sleeping, they may inhale food into their lungs, which can cause coughing, infection of the airways, or aspiration pneumonia.

Mild to moderate weight loss also occurs. When people have significant weight loss, especially older people whose symptoms of dysphagia developed rapidly, doctors consider and usually look for a tumor at the gastroesophageal junction (the place where the esophagus connects to the stomach).

Pickle Juice, Grain Grass and Mastic Gum are sometimes used as natural remedies for Achalasia. These remedies can possibly give some relief from the symptoms produced by this disorder.

Postural adjustments are changes in body and head posture that may be recommended to reduce aspiration into the lungs. Changes in posture may alter the speed and direction of a food or liquid, and protect the airway to help the patient swallow safely. In general, postural adjustments are intended to be short-term treatments that are used to reduce the chances of aspiration. Specific postures include head tilt, head rotation, chin tuck, side lying and head back. Swallow maneuvers address different swallowing problems.

In general, the thicker the viscosity, the slower the liquid moves, which makes it easier to swallow. Typically, the least viscous liquid is used for mild dysphagia. Increasingly thicker liquids are used to manage more severe forms of the condition.

Research shows thickened liquids can cause risk of dehydration. Thickened liquids make patients feel full and they are flavorless, which gives patients little motivation to drink.

Dietary modification is a key part of dysphagia management. Modifying the texture of food may make it safer to swallow. This may include changing the thickness of liquids, chopping or pureeing solid foods. Eating smaller, more frequent meals can be helpful as well. Changing the taste and temperature of food can also make it easier to swallow and more enticing to eat.

Sometimes smaller volumes of food per swallow may help patients to stimulate a swallow response — this is considered a feeding strategy. Muscle relaxants such as nitroglycerin (Nitrostat) or nifedipine (Procardia) can help before eating.

Alzheimer's Disease

This disease was first characterized in 1906 by a German scientist, Dr. Alzheimer. It seems that this is the most common form of dementia in the world now. It seems to start with loss of short-term memory. As the disease progresses there can be loss of orientation, including getting lost, problems with language, mood swings, loss of self-care, loss of motivation, and behavioral issues. There is no cure for the disease although some of the symptoms can be helped somewhat. And yes, Alzheimer's can be a cause of death.

Here are some natural foods that are at least theorized to help prevent the onset of Alzheimer's.

1. Eat spinach, along with other leafy greens such as kale, collard greens, broccoli, turnip and mustard greens. These vegetables offer a wealth of nutrients and are rich in Vitamin A and C. Just six servings a week can make a massive difference in preventing Alzheimer's.

2. Yes, this diet advocates for the consumption of champagne, but not without limitation. Results showed Champagne, Pinot Meunier, and pinot noir grapes produce specific, beneficial phenolics during fermentation. These compounds can alter proteins that are responsible for memory storage in the brain.

3. These superfoods, which include acai berries, strawberries, raspberries, and blueberries are packed with a wealth of antioxidants. According to the Journal of Alzheimer's Disease, they all

reduce the build-up of plaque in the brain, which is believed to be a key factor in the development of Alzheimer's.

4.   Studies show the high concentration of omega-3s, omega-6s, Vitamin E, folate, vitamin B6, and magnesium in almonds, cashews, hazelnuts, peanut, pecans, and walnuts are effective in preventing Alzheimer's.

5.   Coffee and Caffeine While the jury is still out on the health benefits of coffee overall, studies show it may help with Alzheimer's prevention. The stimulant may delay the onset of Alzheimer's in seniors already showing signs of dementia by blocking brain inflammation and, consequently, cognitive decline.

6.   Dark Chocolate Flavonoids in dark chocolate have long been improving the body's circulation and fighting heart disease, but those same flavonoids may also be fighting off dementia.

7.   Turmeric Whether you make a conscious decision to eat a lot more Indian food or simply drink turmeric tea, this root could benefit your mind. Turmeric is a popular natural health choice, and recently, researchers from UCLA

found a combination of vitamin D3 and turmeric can reduce brain plaque associated with Alzheimer's Disease.

8. Cinnamon Numerous animal studies showcase cinnamon's ability to improve memory and cognitive functioning and reduce the build-up of a protein plaque associated with Alzheimer's disease. Cinnamon seems to have such healing potential that even its scent can improve memory, though you should ingest it to enjoy its anti-inflammatory benefits.

9. Tomatoes, carrots, and beets contain enough folate, iron, and vitamin A to help with cognition. Pair these powerhouses with beans, legumes, and whole grains to up your intake of acetylcholine, a vital neurotransmitter that increases brain function.

It won't hurt to eat these nutritious foods anyway. With or without the anti-Alzheimer's benefits. A strong well-fed body can benefit your health in many ways including slowing the progression of degenerative mental disease like Alzheimer's.

Anemia

Anemia is a shortage of red blood cells needed especially to carry oxygen to the cells and their waste products away from the cells. You can get your hemoglobin checked with a regular blood test and it is not a bad idea to do it at least once a year. Men should have a higher hemoglobin level than women and a man should have at least 14 or 15 units of blood. Women should have at least 12 units of blood. Of course, she has to be constantly making new blood to make up for menstrual losses. The hormone that regulated blood production, erythropoietin, is made in the kidneys, although the blood itself is made in the bone marrow. And yes, iron is a requirement to make that blood. If you have kidney difficulties, you might become anemic and make some dietary adjustments or even have a transfusion of blood added.

If you are anemic, your diet should be alkaline predominantly. Eat raw fruits and vegetable that are rich in iron, particularly dark green leafy vegetables such as spinach, alfalfa, watercress, green onions, kale, broccoli, chard, okra, squash, radishes, beets, yams and tomatoes. Bananas are particularly beneficial. Sunflower seeds contain as much easily assimilable iron as liver. Eat whole wheat, buckwheat, beans, soybeans and millet. Avoid caffeine. It interferes with iron absorption.

There is another common anemia called pernicious anemia in which a person cannot digest Vitamin B-12 because they have a deficiency in their stomachs of an intrinsic factor needed for absorption. In that case you might need to have a vitamin B12 injection or possibly let it dissolve as a lozenge under the tongue.

Anxiety

Anxiety is the most common mental disorder in the US. One out 13 people experience the symptoms and many need treatments. It is a feeling of fear, apprehension, unease or agitation when a person senses some kind of danger or threat. It influences the way you think, feel and behave.

All of us feel anxiety sometimes. It is normal and necessary to increase alertness and prepare the person for action. It becomes a disorder when the feelings are overwhelming, occur frequently, last for an extended period or interfere with your ability to function.

Signs that anxiety may be becoming a dangerous condition for you: unable to concentrate, dizziness, shakiness, excessive eating, sleep difficulties, rapid heartbeat, excessive worrying, biting the nails, being unable to act, and unrealistic fears.

What we have here is a brain malfunction. Damage somehow. Maybe a physical jarring of some sort. Maybe a childhood trauma and that has not been resolved. Possibly some physical nerve fibers that are going to the wrong place or not working at all. Very possibly there is a chemical imbalance. People get drugged up for this condition and are able to function, but will possibly never completely heal once they are addicted to the medicinal drugs, either pharmaceutical or herbal.

I wonder how many people are afflicted with this illness because of what they eat and how they eat. Foods have many ingredients. Thousands of different chemicals. I mean actually thousands of different chemicals. Plant material and animal material both have many micro amounts of substances. Don't you think there is a good chance that some of the chemicals are harmful to the brain? I think so. And could be man-made chemicals that have been added to the food. Maybe in the water. Or the air. Who knows?

If the person with anxiety disorder was my patient, I would try to ween him off any drugs he is taking and try to cleanse him inside and out. A fast for a couple of weeks. Just one juice of his choice for the whole time. Colon cleansing also. Come back easy with just raw foods. Organic. Absolutely no animal products. They are loaded with toxins and the person needs to stay clean. Anxiety may be like an allergy to something in the food. Get clean and then become a vegan. And get some good natural therapeutic counselling. Massage. Yoga. Nature. A new life for you. Anxiety-free. Healthy.

Arthritis

The word arthritis means inflammation of a joint. Inflammation means swollen, redness, warmth, soreness, and restricted movement. It is the body's own way of trying to heal itself. A joint should be able to do all of its normal movements, pain-free and for the full range of its motion. The word arthritis has become sort of a catch-all for any condition in the body's structure that is not thoroughly understood for diagnosing or a treatment. "Oh, it must be arthritis". That apparently means it is permanent and really no cure or even a method of partially alleviating it. Except stronger and stronger pain medications. Or just tough it out and it might get better.

There are various types of conditions that are referred to as arthritis. For example, gout is often called gouty arthritis and rheumatism is rheumatoid arthritis. The most common type of arthritis is no doubt osteoarthritis. This is a wear and tear of structures in the joint, often protective membranes around the ends of the bone and the result is the classic bone on bone description. Many people suffer from traumatic arthritis after a certain amount of time passes after an injury or surgery. Tissues in the joint have been injured and are more susceptible to painful inflammation. There is also a type of arthritis from lack of movement and holding a position for a long time, especially while sleeping.

Yes, pain. All arthritis is painful. Painful to move. Painful to put any pressure on the joint that is affected. Rheumatoid arthritis often affects the fingers, palms, wrists joints in the feet and ankles. Those area are very sensitive anyway, even without arthritis. We have a lot of nerve endings in our hands and feet. It seems to be an autoimmune disease where our own white blood cells are attacking tissues in and around the joint with no relief from massage of the rheumatoid joints. Massage is almost always beneficial if a person is in pain, but not for rheumatoid arthritis. Massage can possibly make it worse.

What about exercise? Actually, I think not exercising can bring on inflammation. Stiffness and pain. But keep your exercise moderate. No straining. Get your circulation moving. Strengthen the muscles around your arthritis. You can do it by holding your muscles in a state of contraction without even any movement. How about walking in a pool? And swimming. What could be better than swimming? Maybe using a paddle board.

I like stretching the joints. Get some drainage in there. Hot then cold. Go through all the motions of the joint. Even rheumatoid. Moving the joint around can increase the swelling and bring on a lot of aggravation. No pain no gain? Stretch and drain the joints. It can lead to pain, but it can add to the healing. Otherwise you just become immobile while you await some kind of surgery. Keep stretching. Gentle movements. Increase your range of motion for every joint. Gently.

How about resistance? Then relax and stretch. Open and close the joint. Every movement that you can think of. Just moving cannot hurt you. Back and forth. Circles. Pull on the joint. Compressing it may be difficult, so don't do anything difficult or painful. Don't squeeze. Don't twist the joint. Just try to open it and draw healing into it. All healing is natural. It is passive. We are born being able to heal all-natural problems naturally. Does prayer help? Sure can't hurt.

I like Dr. Airola's recommendations for arthritis and it was one of his specialties. Alternate juice fasts for several weeks with an all vegetarian raw food diet. The vegetarian diet with emphasis on vegetables, particularly potatoes (cooked and raw) and all available greens. Alfalfa is of specific benefit, as is raw potato juice freshly made. Eat alfalfa seeds sprouted daily. Also wheat grass, watercress, yams, celery, parsley, garlic, comfrey and endive. Best fruits for arthritis are bananas, sour cherries, pineapple and apples.

Quart of goat's milk raw or sour. Millet and brown rice are the best grains. Cut a raw potato into thin slices and let it stand in pure water overnight and drink it in the morning. Drink green juice with carrot juice, beet juice, and celery juice and vegetable broth daily to dissolve the accumulations around the joints. Bromelain from pineapples to eliminate swelling and inflammation. Hot and cold showers morning and evening. Massage and acupuncture. Poke berries, comfrey, slippery elm, burdock, and sassafras teas. Water, water, and more water. Especially for gout. Dilute the acid and the crystals. Dilute and dissolve. Water is the great healer.

Asthma

Asthma affects hundreds of millions of people world-wide . Their breathing passages like bronchii, get narrowed, maybe even blocked by mucus, and the patient suffers from shortness of breath and wheezing. Many are children. Many of them come from families with a history of allergies and hay fever. Quite often the person is having an allergic reaction after inhaling substances such as dust, animal dander, cigarette smoke, pollen, mold, smog or other environmental pollutants. Many bronchial spasms can be brought on by non-allergens such as exercise, emotional stress, cold air, viral infections, and medications.

According to Dr. Airola, many asthmatics have an emotional component to their condition. Many have a deep-seated insecurity and an intense need for parental love and protection. When emotional causes are suspected, these must be dealt with before biological and nutritional treatments can be effective.

There is clear relationship between asthma and low blood sugar. A vegetarian diet is best for asthma patients. Lots of garlic, green vegetables and all available fruit, natural unfiltered honey, seeds, nuts, sprouts and whole grains. The diet should include manganese-rich foods such as peas, beans, blueberries, nuts, and buckwheat. Manganese deficiency could be a contributing cause. Also raw foods containing a lot of Vitamin C. The best juices for asthma are lime, comfrey, horseradish and garlic, mixed with carrot juice and red beet juice. Herbal teas, comfrey, mullein, valerian root. Although pollen can be an allergen it can also be used by asthmatics as a remedy, a couple of teaspoons per day.

A noted naprapath, Dr. C. Ford, claims she can relieve the discomfort of asthma by stimulating the middle thoracic vertebrae with quick gentle thrusting, feeling for tightness here and there and working into the resistance.

Cancer

That dreaded word. Can it be treated naturally? There have been many practitioners and many methods. I don't know of anything that works consistently and reliably. Even the establishment medical world fails often. I believe there will be found a cure for cancer someday. They can stop some forms of cancer now, but there are many types of cancer and many of them will eventually kill the patient.

Usually cancer is overgrowth of cells forming tumors that will eventually get in the way of our natural living procedures. Then the tumor has to be removed or you die. And you might die anyway.

They used to think that cancer was caused by an irritant, something in our food or water or in our regular environment. For instance, guys who worked at steel mill coke plants often acquired cancer from the terrible substances released in the process. Probably also many people who lived nearby. But not everyone. Some people have natural genetic defenses and probably are safe from cancer.

Cell division and multiplication is normal for most of the cells in our body. Maybe not nerve cells. We don't know if they can divide. If they could then a lot of nerve damage from injuries could be repaired much easier. Tumors in the brain are not from nerve cells multiplying. The tumors there are from supporting cells called glia that surround the nerve cells.

Every cell has DNA in its nucleus and when the cell divides the DNA divides. The new cells are identical to the original cells, whether they are normal or cancerous. Built in to the DNA of most people are protective gene segments that prevent the cell from dividing out of control and forming a tumor or some type of malignancy. If you did not inherit that protective gene, then you are more susceptible to getting cancer.

An example is the BRAC gene that protects women from breast cancer and ovarian cancer. A woman I knew had inherited a defective BRAC from her mother and she had both of her breasts removed prophylactically so she would not get cancer there. Unfortunately, she did get the cancer in her ovary and died from that.

Chemicals and other irritants can damage your protective genes even if you inherited good ones. That would cause cells to divide out of control and possibly form a tumor. Tumors that spread to surrounding tissues or metastasize to other part of the body are very possibly cancerous. Many tumors do not spread, and they are called benign. Sometimes they need no treatment. Usually they feel smooth and the tumor moves when you shake it. Here are some examples of benign tumors:

Lipomas grow in fat tissue often on arms, back, and neck

Adenomas grow on tissue covering organs like colon polyps

Myomas grow in muscle tissue including in walls of arteries

Nevi called moles and grow on the skin. Fibroids grow in the tissue of the uterus

When the tumor can spread it is called malignant. All the cells in the tumor are defective. They are all the same kind, but very distorted and deranged. If they get in the lymph or blood vessels, they can start new tumors elsewhere. And every cell in that tumor will be the same defective cells that were in the original tumor. For instance, if a lung tumor spreads to the liver, the tumor on the liver will be composed of those same cancerous lung cells. If breast cancer cells spread to a lymph node, the cancerous breast cells are now multiplying in the lymph node.

Yes, it is a terrible disease. It can happen so fast. Before you know it you have many thousands of defective cells growing in your body and each cell is capable of forming a tumor. I know it sounds hopeless. The right idea to is try to prevent the cells from mutating and becoming cancerous to begin with. That is easier said than done, but not impossible.

Here are my suggestions for avoiding cancer:

Do your best to stay away from carcinogenic substances. There didn't use to be cancer and in certain places it is still very rare. Clean environment and clean living. Clean water. Clean air. Clean food. There is some possible natural growth of cancer in our bodies, but usually it has to be stimulated by something.

Can stress cause cancer? I believe during periods of high stress we produce toxic substances. I'm not sure how exactly it works, but I believe the mind sends out a signal somewhere that causes the toxins to be released. The brain is extremely complex and all the many little parts excrete this or that neurochemical. We need stress to stay alive. Just enough. No extra. Many people in the modern world experience way too much stress. There are chemicals released. Maybe for our protection from too much stress. I'm just saying it is possible that these chemicals might affect the DNA in some type of cell and cause mutations to begin. Sort of like a toxin from your environment.

Eating properly seems to me to be the most critical aspect of cancer prevention. It is really hard to completely avoid poisons in our food and who knows if the poisons can cause a cancer to begin? But we have to eat, and all food now is grown with chemicals one way or another. Organic is certainly safer.

Hormones in our food seems very risky to me. I've read studies associating hormones with possibly starting cancer. The meat industry uses a lot of hormones. Some to make the animal grow faster and some to make the animal's muscle be more tender and surrounded with more fat for the taste. Anyway, I am a vegan and I am against all meat consumption. Too much cruelty and the hormone dangers. It is possible in certain places that meat can be purchased that was not in the feedlots and injected with hormones. Many countries don't want American meat imported because they don't want their kids eating all the female hormones that get injected into farm animals. American girls start their periods now at 10 or 11 because of the hormones in the meat and boys are becoming somewhat feminized.

Eat natural foods, mostly raw. With vibrant colors. A large variety. Every day. And some natural juice. You have to work at it a little, but isn't it worth it to never have to go through a battle with cancer? Nourish your body with healthy food. Unprocessed. Natural.

I want to mention about a treatment I saw at a European cancer health spa. The treatment is natural with no surgery or chemical medications. They don't get 100% remission rates. Neither do the high-tech clinics in the United States, but both types of therapy do have some good results. In the European spa, the first thing they do is put the new patient on a fast for a week or two.

One of the body's natural defenses against cancer is called cachexia. The blood chemistry remains fairly normal in cancer because the blood "cannibalizes" some of your own cells to keep the blood normal. Some of the first cells that get attacked by the blood are the cancer cells. The patient starts to lose a lot of weight from the cachexia.

Fasting is similar to cachexia and the fast tries to stimulate the blood to attack the tumor cells. Which often it does. My point in this is I think everyone should do an occasional fast for at least a week. Preferably 10 days. Just water and lots of it. If you have an unusual growth somewhere in your body, it is possible you can "nip it in the bud."

So those are my suggestions. Eat right, avoid stress, no chemicals in your food, air, water or environment, fast occasionally every year. Probably I should add having your colon cleansed every year also.

Here are some of the common cancers attacking people in the United States and other Western countries. Also here are symptoms to watch for.

Basal cell carcinoma and squamous cell carcinomas on the skin. Millions of new cases every year. Unusual growths or marks on your skin.

Breast cancer. new lumps are the most common symptom of breast cancer, but they're not the only one. You should also watch for nipple discharge; any dimpling, pulling in, or retraction of the breast skin or nipples; a persistent rash; and sometimes, pain. Most lumps are benign.

Lung cancer. Early-stage lung cancers typically don't cause symptoms, but people may experience a persistent or worsening cough, coughing up blood, chest pain, and hoarseness.

Prostate cancer. The most common cancer in men. Though early prostate cancer often has no symptoms, in later stages the disease can cause a slow or weak urine stream, blood or semen in urine, and erectile dysfunction.

Colon cancer. symptoms include bowel changes (like diarrhea or constipation) that last longer than a few days, blood in the stool, cramping, and abdominal pain.

Melanoma. can either show up as a new spot or it can arise within an existing mole, look for a mole that has changed in size, shape, or color. It may be suspicious if a mole has multiple colors or unusual colors like red, white, blue, or black Common symptoms include swollen lymph nodes, chills, fatigue, weight loss, a swollen belly, frequent infections,

Bladder cancer. blood in the urine is typically the first sign of bladder cancer, but it may also lead to changes in urinary habits. More advanced cases can cause an inability to urinate, lower back pain, weight loss, and loss of appetite.

Non-Hodgkin Lymphoma. common symptoms include swollen lymph nodes, chills, fatigue, weight loss, a swollen belly, frequent infections,

Kidney cancer. the symptoms may include blood in the urine, low back pain on one side of the body that's not linked to an injury, a lump in the lower back, fatigue, appetite loss, unexplained weight loss.

Uterine cancer. symptom at least three irregular or abnormal bleeding periods in a row.

Thyroid cancer. symptoms like swelling, or pain, or a lump in the neck, hoarseness and voice changes, constant cough, and trouble breathing or swallowing.

CVD Cardio Vascular Disease

According to many current studies, CVD leads to the main cause of death in America and most Western countries. Heart attack and stroke. The three main risk factors that we are told are high blood pressure, smoking, and high levels of blood LDL cholesterol.

Excess cellular debris from natural metabolism in our blood can form deposits of fats and proteins in our arteries. Often the metabolites contain cholesterol. The contributing factor is the fatty acid triglycerides that we eat in our food. We need some, but not so much as many people eat. We have to start thinking constantly being aware of our food intake. Otherwise, you are going to kill yourself eating.

Dietary lipids are usually triglyceride fats. We do need some in our diet. Maybe around 20 grams of dietary fat per day. That is less than an ounce of fat or oil. It carries fat soluble vitamins like A, D, and E and we need it to synthesize some hormones and our phospholipids that carry cholesterol to cells where it is needed. Of course, it is also a source of energy.

Scientists have found that one of the main causes of our arteries getting dangerously narrowed is the proliferation of smooth muscles cells in the walls of the arteries. We need those smooth muscles because they open and close the arteries in response to where the blood is especially needed. For instance , when you are relaxed and digesting your meal, the arteries to your digestive tract will open wider and the arteries to your arms and legs will narrow because we don't need blood there when we are relaxed.

Proliferation means excessive multiplying of those smooth muscle cells and they form like a growth in the arteries. Sort of like cancer of the arteries. What are some of the suspected causes of that proliferation? Presence of high fat levels in the blood, high blood pressure, type A behavior (stress and tension), obesity, physical inactivity, cigarette smoking (related to hydrocarbons and nicotine), diabetes, family incidence, being a male, and increased age.

The degeneration of the arterial wall is called arteriosclerosis. Quite often caused by the proliferation of the muscle cells in the artery. Cancer is proliferation of cells creating tumors. That is sort of like what is happening here. Tumors in the artery. Often it is accompanied by the deposit of calcium salts, so the artery loses its resiliency. It doesn't stretch like it normally should and becomes susceptible to hemorrhagic bleeding when the blood pressure increases with stress or exercise.

Atherosclerosis is a specialized type of arteriosclerosis with accumulation of fats in the inner wall of the artery. This is coupled with the narrowing from the proliferation of the smooth muscle cells. There is an increased susceptibility to clotting and bleeding.

Without that proliferation of the smooth muscle cells, there will be no arteriosclerosis. That is the first step. Forming kind of a tumor in the artery. There are two main possible causes for that proliferation of the smooth muscle cells. Maybe a cellular mutation that causes the cells to start multiplying. That may be the way some cancers begin. Another possibility is if there is an injury to the artery, possibly by a chemical or some blood ingredient. Anyway blood platelets are attracted to the injury and their excretions cause the muscle cells to proliferate.

At the present time we don't know for sure, but researchers are working on it because it is the main cause of death in our society. Some people just seem to be immune to the cell proliferation and just go on living. Some people are susceptible at a younger age and probably will die from a heart attack or stroke. It might be something that you inherit in your genes and it might not. We just don't know yet.

We do know the results of CVD and the smooth muscle proliferation. The artery is narrowed that goes to nourish the heart muscle itself. It could slowly choke off the blood supply to the heart muscle or there could be a blood clot causing a massive shut down of the blood supply. The result is a myocardial infarction. The heart muscle itself begins to die and then actually stops functioning. It results in a heart attack. And if the artery is going to the brain, you could get a stroke. Either way, it is a terrible thing to happen to a person. Time for some serious consideration of your diet.

Cervical Dysplasia (HPV virus)

The HPV virus is a sexually transmitted virus and common now. Its not new, but its prevalence is sort of new. There weren't that many people displaying genital warts in the old days, but there are sure many people now who are infected, often without any symptoms. There are many different strains of the virus. The weaker strains can cause genital warts. That infection can be pretty severe. In the military guys were held down and groups of the warts on the penis were burned off with heat or an acid. Those are the weaker strains that cause the warts. The stronger strains can cause cervical cancer in women.

Yes, guys can give a woman cancer. The cervix is the narrow passageway between the far end of the vagina leading to the uterus. If a woman is infected by the HPV on her cervix, the cells on the cervix can start to change from normal to abnormal and possibly lead to cervical cancer. The cells are obtained in a test called the PAP smear and examined very closely for the growing abnormalities in the cells. That is not exactly the beginning of cancer, but it can lead to cancer. It is possible that your own body can eliminate the defective cervical cells, but it is also possible it will need to be scraped or lasered off. Or even a surgery on the cervix if it is bad enough. If it is not found it can spread throughout the cervix and also cause uterine cancer.

So what can you do prevent this terrible disease. You don't want cervical cancer and you don't want genital warts. Guys might have warts and maybe won't tell you or maybe he doesn't know himself. You have to get some serious testing done to find out if you are a carrier. People used to have indiscriminate sex whenever they felt like it. They can't do that anymore. Way too dangerous. If I was a woman, I would not trust a guy because he is wearing a condom. It can slip off and expose her to her death. If you want to be safe from these and the other sexually transmitted disease you have to get married and never cheat on your partner and that goes for both people. Get tested and married and live your sex life in trusting safety. That is what our parents did for many generations and these diseases were not a problem because they never cheated on their spouses. Get tested and get married. Then you can have sex, but not until then.

Cholesterol

The silent killer. There are no symptoms of high cholesterol levels in your blood. You just die. Drop dead. Heart attack or stroke.

We need cholesterol to stay alive. We make our own. Quite a bit of it. 1000 mg a day in the liver. We need it to hold our cell walls together in every cell in our body. We use it to make bile in our liver and that is used to emulsify fats that we eat. It makes them more easily digested. Without the bile the fat has a tendency to be in large globs, but the bile breaks it into small particles that we can absorb. We need fats in our diet. We also need cholesterol to make Vitamin D and also some of our most important hormones, the steroids and all the sex hormones.

So, what is the problem with cholesterol that leads to atherosclerosis and blockage of some of our most critical arteries? It is used in so many places and we have to carry it around in our blood, so every cell has access to cholesterol. Well, cholesterol itself does not mix well with blood. In our liver, we coat it with proteins so it can transport easily in the blood. These are called lipoproteins.

There are low density lipoproteins (LDL) which are the culprits that deposit cholesterol in plaques in our arteries and interfere with our blood flow especially to the heart and brain. Sometimes the plaque tears loose and becomes part of a blood clot that prevents some of the tiny but critical blood vessels from letting the blood flow through and can lead to the actual heart muscles dying, and in the brain, all sorts of things can go wrong.

Associated with the cells of the inner walls of the arteries are white blood cells called scavenger cells that attack the LDL and the cholesterol inside them deposits in the walls of the arteries. Is it a flaw in the system that the scavenger cells go after the LDL? Well, they don't in everyone. There are some people who can eat almost anything and live easily into their 80's and 90's.

I guess you would say it is an autoimmune disease. The layer of protein that the liver coats the cholesterol with sets off the white blood cells which are part of our immune system. Some people it does, some people it doesn't. We all have different sensors on our white blood cells. Does susceptibility to heart disease and strokes run in families. I think it does.

If people in your family died of heart attacks and strokes, does that mean that you will also? Not necessarily. The person that died may have had a poor diet. No exercise. Some bad luck. They may have had a severe stress that caused a creation of a blood clot that blocked the artery and might not have even had cholesterol plaques. So, you can't say for sure if you are susceptible to a cholesterol caused heart attack or stroke just because someone in your family did.

There is no accurate test at the moment to determine if your LDL's will be attacked by your own scavenger cells. The LDL's themselves will not harm you. They are just floating around in your blood delivering cholesterol to where they may be needed. The whole problem is if your LDL's are attacked by your own immune system and deposits the cholesterol in the artery. There are a lot of auto-immune diseases and this is one of them.

What about the levels of LDL in your blood? Certain levels are considered dangerous indicators of the possibility of having a heart attack. I suppose an abundance of LDL increases your danger, but especially if your white blood cells are going to go after the LDL and the cholesterol will be deposited in the artery. More LDL is more cholesterol is more potential for death. But not necessarily. Not for everyone.

There is a second lipoprotein made in the liver and that is called HDL, high-density lipoprotein. High levels of this lipoprotein are considered beneficial. Their function is to gather up cholesterol when a cell dies and releases it. The HDL is not attacked by the white scavenger blood cells and in fact it can work in conjunction with the scavenger cells. When LDL are attacked, and the cholesterol is released there, it is possible the HDL can pick up the cholesterol and bring it back to the liver for reprocessing, and excess unused cholesterol will be eliminated in the feces. It is natural and safe. So, as it sounds, there should be an optimal balance between LDL and HDL for your good safety.

Can you do anything to affect your LDL and HDL balance? Yes. You can do a lot For one thing, you can cut back on eating meats and dairy that contains a lot of cholesterol.

Fruits and vegetables that contain Vitamin C and Vitamin E have anti-oxidants that slow the susceptibility of the LDL's to the scavenger cells. Excess iron in your blood causes an increase in the

LDL scavenger cell interaction. We need iron, but not in excess. Everything in our bodies works with a balance. Certain drugs increase LDL cholesterol and decrease HDL cholesterol such as progestins, anabolic steroids, and corticosteroids. Avoid these unless absolutely necessary.

Certain foods are effective in reducing the absorption of cholesterol that we eat. Oats, barley and other whole grains, beans, eggplant and any purple produce, okra, nuts, fruits such as apples, grapes, strawberries, and citrus, soy and soy-based foods, foods rich in fiber, olives, olive oil and other unrefined plant oils, especially flaxseed oil, avocados, seeds and real peanut butter. These contain phytosterols which have chemical structures similar to cholesterol and are absorbed in our digestive tract instead of cholesterol which will instead move out in the bowels.

Colonic Irrigation

About 70 years ago or so, Dr. Robert Woods in Gary, Indiana invented a system of thoroughly cleansing the colon comfortably with water running in and then out through a stainless steel proctoscope inserted into the anus.

Over time, a lot of fecal matter accumulates on the walls of the colon. In some cases, so much fecal matter is caked on the walls that only a small amount is able to be excreted. This is especially prevalent when people do not eat enough fiber in their diet. It leads to constipation and impaction of the fecal matter in the colon.

Over the years many methods have been developed and tried to cleanse the colon. Most are substances that are ingested orally and are claimed to cause the fecal matter to be removed from the walls of the colon and often they do work somewhat, but not really enough. And who knows if the ingredients of the cleansers are possibly toxic.

Dr. Woods had worked with cadavers and noticed the huge amounts of fecal matter that some people carried in their colons. Maybe 20 or 30 pounds that allowed only a small passageway through the colon to defecate.

He knew about enemas of course, but they usually only allow cleansing of a small part of the colon. Enemas are sometimes given with a larger pouch holding the water, but even with these, most of the colon is not cleansed. He also had studied the cleansing methods of the swamis in India when they went into bodies of water and drew enough inside them through their anus to thoroughly clean their colons.

I want to briefly mention the different parts of the colon. On the outside are two small sphincter muscles called the anus. One of the sphincters is controlled by the person so it is kept closed when not defecating. Inside of the anus is the rectum where fecal matter is stored getting ready to defecate.

Above the rectum is a curved section called the sigmoid colon then the descending colon going downwards on your left abdomen. Across the middle of the abdomen is the transverse colon and then coming out of the small intestine is the ascending colon. Below the entrance to the ascending colon on your right side is a blind pouch called the cecum with its attached appendix making white blood cells to protect against infection.

Usually the worst impactions of fecal matter occur in the cecum, the ascending colon and transverse colon. For one thing, those areas do not get help from gravity and any fecal movement there requires your colon muscles. The cecum has no outlet with gravity and is where a lot of bacterial toxins accumulate.

Dr. Woods developed his system to clean the entire colon, but especially the impacted areas of the transverse colon, ascending colon, and the cecum.

The proctoscope is sterilized before it is inserted into the anus. There is one tube to send water in and another exit opening to remove the water after it has been used to clean the colon. By using the correct pressure, the right amount of water can even get deep into the transverse, ascending and cecum areas and cleanse those. When the cecum is being cleansed usually the patient experiences a warmth sensation from the poisons and acids being taken out.

Usually the patient lies on one side and is covered with a sheet. The therapist lifts the sheet from behind and inserts the lubricated proctoscope and does the cleansing by controlling the water entering and leaving the colon. The therapist also has a sight glass in the proctoscope to judge the material being washed out, for instance, if it is solid or not.

Some patients may want their own proctoscope and now they make some out of plastic that will only be used on that patient. It is not recommended that a patient receive more than one colonic irrigation in a month. There is a natural flora in the colon and it can be too clean and that is detrimental to the patient's health.

It may take a few treatments right away to clean a severely impacted colon, but then the patient should not be given another one for a while even if they request it. It does feel good while it is happening and then after it is over, the patient has a wonderful feeling, both in their abdomen and their general mental rejuvenation

Crohn's disease

This is a chronic inflammation in the intestines causing extreme diarrhea and abdominal cramping especially on the lower right -hand side of the abdomen. Often it especially affects the ileum, the distal portion of the small intestines where it enters into the cecum in the large intestine. People sometimes think they are having an attack of appendix inflammation, but that is slightly lower. Appendicitis often starts in the navel area and moves to the lower right abdomen and the pain and nausea become much more severe as it moves. High fever often accompanies inflammation of the appendix and it often requires emergency surgery to save the patient's life.

Crohn's is not as acute as appendicitis. Crohn's lasts for a long time and may have flare-up periods, and also periods with none of the symptoms. It is considered to be an auto-immune disease and the symptoms may result in your own immune system mistakenly attacking your own intestinal cells. Why? No one knows for sure, but they think there could be a gene passed to a child to make the person more susceptible to Crohn's. Caucasians seem to be more susceptible and especially Jews.

So what happens? Normally our immune system is on alert for microbes that don't belong in our intestines. Some microbes such as bacteria, fungi, viruses, and a myriad of other little organisms are normal in our system and that is what we call our normal flora. Is it possible that some people develop an immune reaction against their friendly organism and some kind of chemicals are released that cause a toxic reaction. That is one possible cause, but really no definitive cause has yet been determined.

I personally think it caused by our own white cells attacking the cells of the ileum and maybe the cecum and maybe the ileocecal valve. For some inherited reason that we don't understand yet, the cells of ours have external markers on their coats that are similar to markers on a microbe that our immune system fought and maybe defeated, but what our white cells do is make many copies of themselves and are continually on guard if that microbes tries to return.

The white cells "on guard" recognize the markers on our own intestinal cells as belonging to that enemy microbe. It is a mistake. Probably inherited. The intestinal cells probably should not have had those markers that match the microbe, but they do, and our own immune system white blood cells attack our own intestinal cells. Our white cells are nasty fighters and cause our intestinal cells some extreme aggravation.

So the idea is to try and weaken our immune system. Of course, that may leave us open to attacks in other places if we weaken our defenses. That is what happens with immune suppressants, but it can possibly give the Crohn's sufferer some relief. What about more natural self-medications? I personally am not a pill or supplement person, but I do believe in appropriate natural sources. In this case, it has been found that large doses like 2000 IU of vitamin E may have a retarding effect on your immune system. This can be done with your diet. Cold-pressed vegetable oils, wheat germ oil and fresh wheat germ, soybean oil. Scrambled eggs. Sprouted seeds, molasses, sweet potatoes. Green juices from leafy greens, but juiced. We don't want to add much fiber to the det. I think probiotic very fresh yogurt and uncooked sauerkraut juice will help the immune system fight the invading microbes, so maybe our own immune system will not have to be so active. Nobody really knows for sure what is beneficial because nobody really understands exactly what is happening. Those are products I would use during a flare-up, but no guarantees.

Common cold

The common cold is a viral infection of your nose and throat (upper respiratory tract). It's usually harmless. Many types of viruses can cause a common cold. Children younger than six are at greatest risk of colds, but healthy adults can also expect to have two or three colds annually. Most people recover from a common cold in a week or 10 days. Symptoms might last longer in people who smoke.

Symptoms:

Runny or stuffy nose

Sore throat

Cough

Congestion

Slight body aches or a mild headache

Sneezing

Low-grade fever

Generally feeling unwell (malaise)

The discharge from your nose may become thicker and yellow or green in color as a common cold runs its course. This isn't an indication of a bacterial infection.

Causes

Although many types of viruses can cause a common cold, rhinoviruses are the most common culprit.

A cold virus enters your body through your mouth, eyes or nose. The virus can spread through droplets in the air when someone who is sick coughs, sneezes or talks.

It also spreads by hand-to-hand contact with someone who has a cold or by sharing contaminated objects, such as utensils, towels, toys or telephones. If you touch your eyes, nose or mouth after such contact or exposure, you're likely to catch a cold.

Risk factors;

Age. Children younger than six are at greatest risk of colds, especially if they spend time in child-care settings.

Weakened immune system. Having a chronic illness or otherwise weakened immune system increases your risk.

Time of year. Both children and adults are more susceptible to colds in fall and winter, but you can get a cold any time.

Smoking. You're more likely to catch a cold and to have more severe colds if you smoke.

Exposure. If you're around many people, such as at school or on an airplane, you're likely to be exposed to viruses that cause colds.

Prevention

There's no vaccine for the common cold, but you can take common-sense precautions to slow the spread of cold viruses:

Wash your hands. Clean your hands thoroughly and often with soap and water, and teach your children the importance of hand-washing. If soap and water aren't available, use an alcohol-based hand sanitizer.

Disinfect your stuff. Clean kitchen and bathroom countertops with disinfectant, especially when someone in your family has a cold. Wash children's toys periodically.

Use tissues. Sneeze and cough into tissues. Discard used tissues right away, then wash your hands carefully.

Teach children to sneeze or cough into the bend of their elbow when they don't have a tissue. That way they cover their mouths without using their hands.

Don't share. Don't share drinking glasses or utensils with other family members. Use your own glass or disposable cups when you or someone else is sick. Label the cup or glass with the name of the person with the cold.

Steer clear of colds. Avoid close contact with anyone who has a cold.

Choose your child care center wisely. Look for a child care setting with good hygiene practices and clear policies about keeping sick children at home.

Take care of yourself. Eating well, getting exercise and enough sleep, and managing stress might help you keep colds at bay.

Cystic Fibrosis

Cystic fibrosis is a hereditary disease that affects the lungs and digestive system. The body produces thick and sticky mucus that can clog the lungs and obstruct the pancreas.

Cystic fibrosis (CF) can be life-threatening, and people with the condition tend to have a shorter-than-normal life span.

Sixty years ago, many children with CF died before reaching elementary school age. However, advances in treatment mean that people with CF often live into their 30s, 40s, and beyond. There is currently no cure for CF. It affects some 30,000 people in the United States with around 1,000 new cases diagnosed each year. Of these new diagnoses, 75 percent are made in children under the age of 2 years. How sad when a child that young has such a debilitating illness.

Mucus is a slippery substance that lubricates and protects the linings of the airways, digestive system, reproductive system, and other organs and tissues. In people with cystic fibrosis, the body produces mucus that is abnormally thick and sticky. This abnormal mucus can clog the airways, leading to severe problems with breathing and bacterial infections in the lungs. These infections cause chronic coughing, wheezing, and inflammation. Over time, mucus buildup and infections result in permanent lung damage, including the formation of scar tissue (fibrosis) and cysts in the lungs.

Most people with cystic fibrosis also have digestive problems. that result from a buildup of thick, sticky mucus in the pancreas. The pancreas is an organ that produces insulin (a hormone that helps control blood sugar levels). It also makes enzymes that help digest food. In people with cystic fibrosis, mucus often damages the pancreas, impairing its ability to produce insulin and digestive enzymes. Problems with digestion can lead to diarrhea, malnutrition, poor growth, and weight loss.

Cystic fibrosis used to be considered a fatal disease of childhood. With improved treatments and better ways to manage the disease, many people with cystic fibrosis now live well into adulthood. Adults with cystic fibrosis experience health problems affecting the respiratory, digestive, and reproductive systems.

Most men with cystic fibrosis are unable to father children (infertile) unless they undergo fertility treatment. Women with cystic fibrosis may experience complications in pregnancy.

Depression

Depression has certainly become a prevalent disorder in our society. Many scientists think there is a close correlation between mental depression and dietary deficiencies. They can sort of understand the chemistry of depression, but really it will be a long time before they have it down in detail. Anyway, they know chemical deficiencies are probably involved and that leads back to dietary deficiencies.

I am not able to point out a particular part of a person's diet that can lead to depression. Nobody knows that yet. Nutritional psychiatrists work with strengthening their patient's diet in general. Make sure everything is covered I your diet. All the nutrients without overdoing anything. Lots of fruits and vegetables, nuts and whole grains and seeds, fresh juices, cold-pressed olive oil. Everything else is of questionable value in the maintenance of physical and mental health.

Let me list some of the possible symptoms of a developing condition of depression. If you have some of these, you may have the start of a problem. You don't have to run right out and get medicated up. First do a fast and redo your diet and see if that helps.

Here are the indicators. Substance abuse, feelings of failure, unexpected weight loss, unusual joint pain, thoughts of suicide, long-lasting general sadness, dwelling on unpleasant thoughts, reclusiveness, getting slower, sleep difficulties, need to control, loss of concentration, forgetfulness, fatigue, low self-esteem, neglecting your appearance and hygiene, spending a lot of time worrying.

There are many anti-depressant medications available, but I have to wonder if you might become dependent on them and then into a progression of stronger medications. It seems to me that a person should always try the mildest palliative first and that would be to improve your diet and maybe make some changes in your lifestyle. Maybe some counselling without prescriptions.

There is no miracle cure that I know of. No herb or pill or supplement or food. Nothing that works for sure. What you want is to live your life in a general state of happiness. Right? That begins with a good diet. Lots of green leaves. Cooked and raw. A myriad of colorful foods every day. That's how you make sure all your needs are covered. Colors in foods are important and yes, white is a color. You don't need meat or dairy products. Everything you could possibly need can be found in fruits and vegetables. And don't forget berries.

Be patient. Give nature time to heal you. Your health is forever. Take your time. Do it right. Dwell on feeling better. Every day smile at someone or at many people. Smile in a mirror. And feel your happiness surging through your mind. Fell happiness in every part of your body. Be glad for all the wonderful blessings you have. Yell out loud, "thank you for making me who I am." Every day you will be better than you were. A lifetime of positive growth. Appreciation for who you are. Contributing to the betterment of the Earth and all of life. It all starts with eating properly. Nutrition for your body and your mind.

Diabetes and Brewer's Yeast

Offenbacher and Sunyer, examined 24 elderly subjects, who were fed daily for 8 weeks with brewers' yeast as a source for GTF (glucose tolerance factor). They found a considerable improvement in glucose tolerance and insulin sensitivity, and a reduction of total fats in these patients.

Grant and McMullen treated 37 type 2 diabetics for 7 weeks, in a double-blind study, with either brewers' yeast as a source of GTF, or a placebo. Supplementation of brewers' yeast significantly decreased HbA1c and increased HDL cholesterol in the treated group.

Elwood supplemented 27 subjects with brewers' yeast. He found that total circulating cholesterol was significantly reduced, and the HDL levels were significantly increased with brewers' yeast.

Riales reported that human subjects receiving 7g of brewers' yeast for 6 weeks had a significant decrease in serum LDL and an increase in HDL cholesterol.

Since GTF is supposed to be essential for normal glucose tolerance in mammals, and as muscle tissue consumes a major part of blood glucose, it is most important to assess the effect of GTF on muscle tissue. The effect of GTF obtained from brewer's yeast extract increased the rate of glucose transport into cells, 2 to 2.5 fold, in the absence of insulin.

The exact composition and structure of GTF from Brewer's yeast is still obscure, but it has been suggested that it is a small molecule containing chromium and some amino acids. There are other active components, but the exact structure is not known yet.

Diabetes and GTF

There are over 400 million people afflicted with diabetes in the world. It is found somewhat in third world countries, but in the wealthier over-eating countries, it is the third leading cause of death. World medical expenditures on diabetes is approaching 500 billion dollars a year. The disease is generally divided into two major types: Insulin Dependent Diabetes Mellitus (IDDM, or type 1), and Non Insulin Dependent Diabetes Mellitus (NIDDM, or type 2 DM).

Diabetes basically results from an insulin malfunction and subsequent large amount of glucose accumulation in the body. Both forms are devastating with respect to their complications. Insulin is released from the pancreas when we eat food containing glucose and the insulin functions by assisting the sugars to be taken into cells, especially muscle cells to be used for energy. Not enough insulin and the glucose sugar begins to accumulate in the blood.

The Type I diabetes usually appears during youth. It is an auto-immune disease in which our own white blood cells destroy the beta cells in the pancreas which make our insulin. That's why the Type I patients are dependent on an external source of the insulin. The type II disease usually comes later in life and some of the associated factors are obesity, high blood pressure, over-eating , especially sugars and refined starches like white flour, and a sedentary lifestyle. Those are causes that can start the insidious destruction of having too much sugar in our blood.

People with diabetes have a 25-fold increase in the risk of blindness, a 20-fold increase in the risk of kidney failure, a 20-fold increase in the risk of amputation as a result of gangrene and a 2 to 6-fold increase in the risk of coronary heart disease and brain damage from blood blockage. In general, life expectancy for a person with diabetes is decreased by one-third.

Diabetes Insulin Resistance

In this condition, the body does not respond to insulin as it should. Sometimes it is called impaired glucose tolerance. It can possibly lead to type 2 diabetes, heart disease and vascular disease. It can be associated with obesity, high blood pressure and high blood triglycerides.

Insulin activates a protein, GLUT4, to bind to glucose and allows it into the muscle cells especially, so that the glucose can be used for energy. After we eat, the pancreas sends insulin into the blood to be carried to the muscles. The insulin level quickly declines so that we do not become hypoglycemic, too low in sugar. Everything works by levels and balances. Just enough of everything.

With insulin resistance, the body does not respond to the insulin from the pancreas so excess glucose has higher than normal levels in the blood. This causes the release of more insulin from the pancreas and the condition is called hyperinsulinemia.

Pre-diabetes and metabolic syndrome, which may develop in association with insulin resistance, can cause several signs and symptoms, including:

- Frequent urination
- Excessive thirst
- Dark patches on the groin, armpits, or back of the neck that are known as acanthosis nigricans
- Weight gain

- High triglyceride levels and low HDL (good cholesterol)
- High blood pressure
- Heart disease

Here are three tests to possibly determine if you are insulin resistant.

Fasting blood glucose test: A fasting blood glucose level between 100 mg/dl and 125 mg/dl is typical of those who are insulin resistant.

Oral glucose tolerance test: This test requires that you abstain from eating and drinking for 12 hours before the test. You will have your blood sugar checked, drink a sugary fluid, and have your blood glucose tested again after time has passed. In general, blood glucose over 140 mg/dl after three hours is suggestive of pre-diabetes or diabetes. There may be a correlation between high blood glucose levels and insulin resistance.

Hemoglobin A1C test: This test measures your average glucose level over the past two to three months. A normal level is between 4 percent and 5.6 percent; a level between 5.7 percent and 6.4 percent is consistent with prediabetes and insulin resistance.

Insulin resistance is becoming more common, and about 10 percent of young adults fit the criteria and 44 percent of adults in the over-60 age group do so as well. Insulin resistance is considered a very early sign that you could be at risk for diabetes. Three obvious treatment regimens are weight loss, exercise, and a diet composed mostly, of fruits, vegetables, nuts, and whole grains

Diabetes and fructose

Table sugar is called sucrose and it is a combination of fructose and glucose, theoretically in a 50/50 ratio. Our digestive system has an enzyme that breaks the two sugars apart, then the glucose goes into the blood and is carried to the muscles, the brain, and other tissues that need the glucose for their energy. The fructose goes to the liver and is often turned into triglyceride fat that we store in our adipose tissue.

Because fructose does not increase blood glucose and does not require insulin, individuals with diabetes can often tolerate it better than other sugars. In fact, studies show that small amounts of oral fructose may actually improve sugar control in people with diabetes. Especially if the source of the fructose is natural fruits and vegetables.

Excess body fat results when people do not balance their energy input with energy output. Extra calories may come from any caloric nutrient—proteins, fats, alcohol and carbohydrates including starches and sugars such as fructose. Lack of physical activity plays a significant role in promoting body fat accumulation and development of obesity.

Some researchers have speculated that fructose may not produce feeling of fullness as other carbohydrates because it does not stimulate insulin and leptin secretion nor suppress ghrelin production—all hormones that help to regulate hunger and food intake. However, it is important to note that this speculation is based on preliminary research that tested fructose levels at least three to four times higher than the average amount consumed by Americans. Further, very few Americans ever consume fructose in isolation, but rather in combination with glucose. An example is high fructose corn syrup, HFCS.

Usually HFCS is 55% fructose and 45% glucose and regular table sugar is 50% each. So there is really not enough difference to claim any therapeutic value to HFCS. The reason it is added to so many processed foods is not because it is healthier for people. It is because it sweetens the food much cheaper than sugar. After all, the Midwest is almost covered with corn and lots of it can be made into HFCS much cheaper than refining sugar cane and sugar beets into table sugar.

There have been many studies relating America's increasing usage of HFCS to our increased obesity and increased Diabetes Type 2. Also, they have tried to relate it to heart disease and types of cancer. But it doesn't work. During the period of Americans using large amounts of HFCS, Americans overeat period. And a lot of junk food. High calorie stuff. We eat more calories than we use in energy and the leftover energy is stored as fat. Triglycerides made in the liver and stored in our adipose tissue. It can be from sugar or it can be from HFCS. They both result in excess calories. If we are sedentary, meaning sitting too much, it is going to become fat. Insulin resistance. Metabolic syndrome and then diabetes.

There is no proof that fructose consumption has any beneficial effects on diabetes, neither established or developing , and no proof that fructose increases the severity of the disease. Like anything that we consume, the "dose" is what counts. Extreme fructose consumption is sure to cause problems somewhere, beginning in the liver. Eat it in moderation in a natural form like in fruits and vegetables and there will be no adverse effects. Fructose is a totally natural component of many foods. Eat them without concern and that is even if you are diabetic.

If you are eating a lot of high fructose corn syrup, that means you are eating way too much highly processed food. Sure, it is convenient. Open it and eat. Or drink. Yes, a lot of it is in pop or juices. I personally do not like the taste of any processed food. So not is it only unhealthy to eat, it is not even enjoyable to me. You can break your bad habit of eating that stuff and start eating natural whole foods with no additives.

Diabetes Home Remedy

Activity. Burn off that glucose. Use your muscles and use your mind. Stop watching television or at least cut way back on viewing time. Television time actually uses less energy that sleeping. I don't know exactly how that works. It is something about all the info is coming in to your passive brain with no real responsiveness.

Eat a lot of alkaline foods because diabetics often have over acidity in the blood. So eat lots of vegetables and fruits. Yes, fruits. Especially grapefruits and bananas.

Cucumbers, green beans, artichokes, avocados, and garlic are beneficial. And lots of nuts.

Try to make 80% of your diet raw food. It is stimulating to your pancreas to secrete insulin.

Diabetics need to eat natural, unrefined complex carbohydrates. Things that enter your blood slowly. Like whole grains, especially millet, oats, buckwheat, brown rice, quinoa, barley, spelt, bulgur, and amaranth. Eat like that and live to be 100. No sugar or white flour, or salt.

Many small meals in a day. No overeating. No large meals. Diabetes is unknown in countries where people cannot afford to overeat. Most diabetics are overweight. So try to lose weight. Overeating most anything will eventually turn into fat. Eating too much food taxes the pancreas and interferes with normal insulin production.

Avoid all nervous stress. Find ways to relax. Maybe some kind of exercise or hobby or friends. Laugh ad smile. Really smile. Massage is good even doing yourself with a dry brush. Keeping your circulation working well is critical for diabetics.

Your water is important. Diabetes is prevalent in areas with soft water. Better to drink hard water with minerals like chromium and manganese. Chromium aids in metabolism of excess glucose in your blood. You don't need a lot. Not large supplements. Just a little in your water will help. They sell water with chromium. Another good source of chromium is brewer's yeast. It helps control that excess sugar.

Fresh, raw, natural cucumber juice contains a hormone-like chemical that nourishes the beta cells of the pancreas that make the insulin. Also juices from onions and garlic. And of course, find a way to get fresh stringbean juice. For some reason, it stimulates insulin production. And make tea from the pods of stringbeans.

Cactus pads have a natural chemical similar to insulin and tea from a cactus called Sinita Organo is said to have insulin-like qualities.

If you are already into treatment for diabetes with heavy meds, you cannot just stop them. You can ease the natural treatment in and eventually ease the medications out. Slowly. Little by little. Monitor your progress. If your diabetes is not severe, you might be able to eliminate drugs and control the diabetes naturally. It is possible.

Dupuytren's contracture

There is a diseased growth of connective tissue from the inside of the palm towards the little finger or maybe more fingers. It is strong like scar tissue and impossible for the afflicted person to straighten their fingers back to their open position. Mostly in people from Northern European descent. Sometimes it runs in families. Usually affects older men. Over 50 years old. The actual cause is unknown.

There are several types of surgeries available for a patient, but the problem is the condition has a tendency to recur. It is not actually a disease of the connective tissue of the hand, it is a systemic disease that is not cured by the surgery. Some things that go wrong, we just have to learn to live with. There is no pain, just the disability of some hand uses.

Someday a scientist will figure this disease out and work out a way to help a patient with the disease. Eliminate the systemic cause of the disease and then there would be a method to have a lasting improvement. I read that in Norway, 30% of older men are afflicted with this condition. Something goes wrong. No one knows why or even what goes wrong. We just know the results. The little finger moves toward the palm because of an unnatural growth of connective tissue. Is it an autoimmune disease? I think so, but I don't know the progress or cause of the affliction. Nobody knows yet.

Eczema

Eczema is a term for several different types of skin swelling. Eczema is also called dermatitis. Most types cause dry, itchy skin and rashes on the face, inside the elbows and behind the knees, and on the hands and feet. Scratching the skin can cause it to turn red, and to swell and itch even more.

Eczema is a widespread disease and affects 30 million people in the US alone. It is most common for babies and children to develop eczema on their face (especially the cheeks and chin), but it can appear anywhere on the body and symptoms may be different from one child to the next. More often than not, eczema goes away as a child grows older, though some children will continue to experience eczema into adulthood. Adults can develop eczema, too, even if they never had it as a child.

Symptoms are red, scaly areas, small, rough bumps, thick, leathery patches, bumps that leak fluid and crust over.

If you have dark skin, the affected area might be lighter or darker.

There are many natural therapies for eczema.

Coconut oil.

Sunflower oil.

Topical vitamin B12.

Training the mind to relax

Massage.

Colloidal oatmeal is made from finely-ground oats.

Evening primrose oil.

Witch hazel.

Calendula cream.

Acupuncture and acupressure.

While there is no cure for eczema, there are many treatments to help manage the symptoms. Since dry skin leads to itchiness and inflammation, the goal of treatment is to find the best cream or ointment that will keep your skin moisturized (not dry) and lessen inflammation. ... Wet compresses to soothe and hydrate skin.

Fibroids

Uterine fibroids are very common non-cancerous growths (tumors) of the uterus. Approximately 40 percent of Caucasian women and 60 percent of African American women over the age of 35 will develop fibroids in their lifetime. Uterine fibroids have no size limitation. They can often be as large as a grapefruit. While these are benign (non-cancerous) tumors, they do cause many problems. Many of these symptoms are related to the pressure caused by these abnormal masses. Overall, the symptoms can be very debilitating.

Women suffering from the symptoms of uterine fibroids often find their lives very compromised. As a result, it is a high priority to seek appropriate treatment. Treatment options vary from newer minimally invasive solutions (uterine fibroid embolization) to traditional surgery.

Common Uterine Fibroid Symptoms Include:

Heavy or prolonged bleeding

This can lead to dangerous anemia, sometimes requiring blood transfusion.

Very painful menstrual period

Pelvic pain and pressure

Back pain

Pain during intercourse (dyspareunia)

Bladder pressure, causing frequent urination

Constipation, causing bowel pressure and pain

Abdominal bloating

Although researchers continue to study the causes of fibroid tumors, little scientific evidence is available on how to prevent them. Preventing uterine fibroids may not be possible, but only a small percentage of these tumors require treatment. But, by making healthy lifestyle choices, such as maintaining a normal weight and eating fruits and vegetables, you may be able to decrease your fibroids.

uterine fibroids aren't associated with an increased risk of uterine cancer and almost never develop into cancer. Fibroids range in size from seedlings, undetectable by the human eye, to bulky masses that can distort and enlarge the uterus. You can have a single fibroid or multiple ones. In extreme cases, multiple fibroids can expand the uterus so much that it reaches the rib cage. Uterine fibroids develop from a stem cell in the smooth muscular tissue of the uterus (myometrium). A single cell divides repeatedly, eventually creating a firm, rubbery mass distinct from nearby tissue. The growth patterns of uterine fibroids vary — they may grow slowly or rapidly, or they may remain the same size. Some fibroids go through growth spurts, and some may shrink on their own.

Heredity. If your mother or sister had fibroids, you're at increased risk of developing them. Black women are more likely to have fibroids than women of other racial groups. In addition, black women have fibroids at younger ages, and they're also likely to have more or larger fibroids. Onset of menstruation at an early age; use of birth control; obesity; a vitamin D deficiency; having a diet higher in red meat and lower in green vegetables, fruit and dairy; and drinking alcohol, including beer, appear to increase your risk of developing fibroids.

Natural treatment of fibroids

Fibroids typically grow slowly or not at all. In many cases, they shrink on their own, especially after menopause. You may not need treatment unless you're bothered by symptoms.

Fibroids may be treated with ultrasound therapy. At-home care, diet changes, and natural remedies may help treat fibroids and relieve symptoms.

Weight loss

A clinical study in China showed that obesity and excess weight increased the risk for uterine fibroids. This happens because fat cells make high amounts of estrogen. Losing weight may help prevent or reduce the size of fibroids.

Foods to avoid

According to clinical studies, eating too much red meat increases your risk of uterine fibroids. Drinking alcohol also increases your risk. Eating excess refined carbohydrates and sugary foods may trigger or worsen fibroids. These foods raise blood sugar levels. This causes your body to produce too much insulin hormone. Avoid or restrict simple refined carbohydrates like: white rice, pasta, and flour, soda and other sugary drinks, corn syrup, boxed cereals, baked goods (cakes, cookies, doughnuts),potato chips, crackers

Foods to eat`

Fiber-rich unprocessed foods. Brightly colored foods such as fruits and vegetables also help reduce inflammation and lower your risk for fibroids. Add these whole foods to your daily diet: raw and cooked vegetables and fruit, dried fruit, whole grains, brown rice, lentils and beans, whole grain bread and pasta , couscous, quinoa, green tea

Fibromyalgia

It affects 5 million men and women in the US alone. It is chronic, long-lasting pain affecting various parts of the body. The pain seems to be a deep muscle pain with morning stiffness. The pain can radiate away from a central area and causes extreme tenderness to being touched there. Certain points are often under the surface of the skin, not in areas of deep pain. It's the tissue around the muscles and joints that hurts rather than the joints themselves.

Along with pain-related symptoms, people living with fibromyalgia often experience the following symptoms and co-conditions. Problems sleeping, fatigue, difficulty thinking clearly (also known as "fibro fog" among patients), difficulty performing everyday tasks, stress and anxiety, depression, migraine headaches, numbness, and tingling in hands, arms, feet, and legs. There can also be irritable bowel syndrome and difficulty urinating associated with fibromyalgia.

The exact cause of fibromyalgia is unknown, however, it is suspected to possibly be an autoimmune disease. People suffering from other autoimmune disorders such as rheumatoid arthritis are more likely to develop fibromyalgia. There is also some evidence to suggest that certain illnesses or infections can act as a trigger. The genes you inherit from your parents may increase the likelihood of developing fibromyalgia. Physical and emotional trauma have also been linked to fibromyalgia.

Researchers believe that fibromyalgia amplifies painful sensations by affecting the way your brain processes pain signals. Some say it's like having the flu. Some compare it to working long hours and missing a lot of sleep. You may feel too tired to exercise or more tired after a workout. Simple things such as grocery shopping or cooking dinner could wipe you out. Starting a project such as folding clothes or ironing could seem like too much effort. You might even be too tired for sex.

About two-thirds of people with fibromyalgia often have belly pain, gas, and bloating and feel like throwing up. They can also have constipation and diarrhea. Many have acid reflux or gastroesophageal reflux disease (GERD), too. Women with fibromyalgia may have unusually painful menstrual cramps, often for years, along with their other symptoms. Some people experience Restless Legs Syndrome which usually affects your feet and legs below your knees. It may hurt, but more often it feels like you need to move your legs to try to make them comfortable. It's especially bothersome at night because it can keep you from sleeping.

It certainly is possible that fibromyalgia can be caused by stealth organism that hide in your cells, sort of like in Lyme disease. These can be very disruptive to your immune system and add a stress to your body that can result in the symptoms of fibromyalgia. Try natural therapies such as heat, soaking in hot water, steam baths, whirlpools, massage, relaxation therapies such as yoga and meditation. Don't be skeptical. These things work.

Many people have been abusing their bodies eating processed foods and meat and sugar. Try revising your diet to natural fruits and vegetables, seeds and grains. Stimulate your immune system in a good way and let your body heal itself. It may take a while, but it is certainly worth trying.

Fibromyalgia is a natural disorder because we don't know anything positively specific that causes it. It definitely could be some kind of microorganism especially one that hides in cells throughout your body. They have meds to give pain relief of your system and they definitely might work, but if you want permanent relief of the disorder, the best chance is with your own body bringing about a cure. It is your best chance for relief permanently.

Diversify. Beyond vegetables, your diet should be proportionally divided among other natural food sources. The more diverse your diet, the closer you will come to fulfilling dietary requirements for optimal wellness.

Hydration is key to keeping your body in top working condition, whether you have fibromyalgia or not. It helps to nourish your cells, detox the body, aid in digestion, control inflammation, and so much more.

This includes drinking eight glasses of water per day, yes, but also eating hydrating foods. Water from food is more alkalized (optimal for absorption) and, in some cases, cleaner than the water you can get from your tap. Good options are apples, berries, cucumbers, watermelon, and romaine lettuce.

Up your omega-3 fatty acid intake. It's a great way to stave off inflammation caused by fibromyalgia. It also helps alleviate oxidative stress, aids in cognitive function, and supports cardiovascular health. To get more omega-3s, flaxseeds, walnuts, and algae are good vegetarian options.

If you have significant digestive dysfunction, restrict your diet to foods that are easily digested and don't ignite food sensitivity reactions. This isn't necessarily forever: many foods can be added back in once healing occurs.

Gout

So what about gout? You probably know someone who suffers from gout attacks, at least occasionally. Men more than women. Excess weight is a factor. Maybe shoes that don't fit right. I think old injuries can flare up. One of the big problems is malfunctioning of the kidneys. They are a system of filters for the blood and those filters can be damaged by high blood pressure, maybe diabetes, maybe trouble with the prostate that can cause the urine to back up and actually kill some of the filtering cells called nephrons.

There is a chemical in our food called purines and when it breaks down in the body eventually it forms uric acid and is hopefully excreted through the urinary system. If there is an excess of uric acids it forms very sharp crystals that attach to our joints, usually in the feet, maybe because the natural tendency is for particles to go lower from gravity. It can be pretty painful and the attack is called gout.

Scientists have tried to associate the condition with a family tendency. It could be a genetic predisposition for something to go wrong with the natural uric acid disposal system or it is possible that the people in the same family might have similar eating patterns. Whatever has gone wrong, there is more uric acid floating around in the blood than is normal for the kidneys to cleanse and the crystals form and find a place to really be irritating to the person. Sometimes being able to even walk can become difficult. Luckily, the attacks seem to come and go.

Well since the chemicals that form the uric acid are purines, it makes sense to restrict the intake of purines in our diet, especially if there is any indication that your uric acid levels are higher than normal. This can be determined by a simple blood test.

I think food can be classified into high purine, medium purine, and low purine. I personally don't see any reason for anyone to consume high purine foods, except for possible taste and maybe some gluttony. They include internal organ meats, such as brains, liver, kidneys, and heart, shellfish, anchovies, mackerel, sardines, herring, scallops, wild game, and beer is loaded with purines because of the yeast.

Foods that contain a moderate amount of purines include beef, pork, poultry, fish and seafood, asparagus, cauliflower, spinach, mushrooms, green peas, lentils, dried peas, beans, peanuts, oatmeal, wheat bran and wheat germ. If your uric acid level is high, use these foods sparingly.

Naturally there will be many foods that interfere with the production of uric acid. Some of them neutralize the acidity of the uric acid ad some actually can help prevent the uric acid from forming crystals. I am not going to go into the actual chemical reactions they are involved with, but try some of the following blueberries, cherries, strawberries, cranberries, olives and olive oil, flaxseed and the oil, pinto beans, dark chocolate, apples and apple cider vinegar, high-fiber foods, vegetable juices, especially with carrot juice, lime, bananas, cucumbers, broccoli, green tea, and large amounts of water. At least 8 glasses every day.

HIV (AIDS)

This virus appeared on the scene about 50 years ago or so. It was a whole new game because it is incurable and very likely may cause death, and it is a horrible way to die. The patient loses part of his immune system to the virus and without his T-cells that recognize invaders, the patient becomes susceptible to other diseases that can't be stopped. Well, medical science has made big advances in combatting AIDS, but it is still the most feared of sexually transmitted diseases. Actually, it can be transmitted without sex. Through blood mixing with another person's blood. That means drug needle sharing becomes high risk. Transfusions were dangerous at one time, but now the testing for the virus has made the blood supply safe.

It is likely that the virus can live in sexual fluids, but it is usually not passed by vaginal intercourse because the vaginal tissues are elastic to an extent and usually don't tear so there would be less chance of mixing semen and blood. There is a much greater chance of infection through anal intercourse because the anus is more likely to tear and the semen would mix with the receiving person's blood. In that case, there is a good chance that the HIV virus will be transferred and will lead to AIDS. It takes a while for the AIDS to be developed in the person's body. It might have been prevented if they had used a condom, but that is not for sure. Condoms tear and are purposefully removed sometimes.

Does the HIV virus live in saliva? It is possible it can live in most any fluids or excretions. If a person was having oral sex and was HIV positive, his semen might come in contact with open sores.

Does the HIV virus live in saliva? It is possible it can live in most any fluids or excretions. If a person was having oral sex and was HIV positive, his semen might come in contact with open sores in the mouth and pass the virus that way. It is not likely, but it is possible. It has to get in a person's blood stream. You could take HIV virus and rub it on your skin and you will not be infected unless there was some places where the skin is torn, maybe near the fingernails. What about kissing? It is unlikely, but possible. It usually has to be blood to blood or semen to blood. Can a person who is infected with HIV ever live a normal life again? They would have to always be aware of their condition and take proper precautions. Does the HIV virus live in saliva? It is possible it can live in most any fluids or excretions. If a person was having oral sex and was HIV positive, his semen might come in contact with open sores in the mouth and pass the virus that way. It is not likely, but it is possible. It has to get in a person's blood stream. You could take HIV virus and rub it on your skin and you will not be infected unless there was some places where the skin is torn, maybe near the fingernails. What about kissing? It is unlikely, but possible. It usually has to be blood to blood or semen to blood. Can a person who is infected with HIV ever live a normal life again? They would have to always be aware of their condition and take proper precautions.

Leptin resistance and obesity

Leptin is a hormone messenger produced by our adipose fat cells. So the more fat you have, the more leptin is made and enters the bloodstream and is carried to a part of the brain called the hypothalamus which measures the amount of leptin and if it is high enough, it shuts off our feelings of hunger. We don't need to eat anymore. Satiety. It over-rules the signals from the ghrelin hormone made in the stomach that causes us to feel hunger.

A high leptin level also stimulates us to burn more energy. Even when we are resting. That is because the hypothalamus sends a signal to our pituitary gland that sends a signal to the thyroid gland to release more thyroid hormone which increases our metabolism throughout the body. We burn more energy and at least theoretically, we will lose some weight.

It is like a feedback system. Negative feedback. If there is a lot of leptin given off by our very plump fat cells, then we don't have hunger. That is natural. If leptin levels are lower because we don't have as much fat, then we do have hunger. Our brain thinks we are starving and puts some heavy pressure on us to find food and eat it. Right away. And a lot of it.

We get very hungry and it is difficult to fight off that feeling. That's why many people who lose weight on a diet, regain it again. We have less fat after the diet and less leptin is sent to the brain, and so our body craves food. If our leptin is low from less fat, we also conserve our energy by not releasing as much thyroid hormone and don't burn the fat. Just slow everything down. It is like our natural instinct to prevent starvation and deep instincts like that have a strong control on our minds.

Scientists suspect there is a condition called leptin resistance that could contribute to obesity. Even if you have an abundance of fat and you are producing a lot of leptin, if the hypothalamus wrongly interprets your high leptin levels as low, your brain is stimulated to go into the starvation mode, and we need more food and seek it and eat it and we also reduce our energy being burned. In other words, the fat should normally get used up for energy, but instead we eat more and gain more fat in our cells. Just the opposite of what high eptin levels usually accomplish. People can try to resist the brain's call for more food, but it is very difficult. It is also very difficult to lose weight if we are not burning a lot of energy.

So leptin resistance causes the hypothalamus to make a mistake in measuring the amount of leptin. Even though you have a lot of fat your brain is fooled into calling for more food. Nobody knows for sure what causes this leptin resistance. I think maybe the amount of leptin in the blood of obese people overwhelms the sensors in the hypothalamus and the feedback system shuts off.

Other scientists now think there is actually a disease process going on and the hypothalamus is impeded by being inflamed from the high leptin levels or from high amounts of triglycerides in the blood. Nobody knows for sure what causes the malfunction, and nobody knows for sure if there is a malfunction, but it a good explanation for increased obesity.

Does it do any good to eat foods containing the actual leptin hormone molecule. Or supplements with leptin powder or pills? It might help. It won't hurt to try it, although if you are obese you probably do not have a shortage of leptin in your blood. Probably you already have an excess and your hypothalamus is resistant to it. But it is worth trying. One problem is that leptin is a protein and will probably be digested into its component amino acids in your stomach, so I am skeptical as to the efficacy of the supplements or leptin containing food items. It is possible, though unlikely, that your fat tissue is not producing enough leptin.

Anyway, it is doubtful that any leptin can get past the stomach's digestive juices intact and still usable. It has to be made in the fat cells. Just eat natural, whole foods. Avoid processed food, extra fats, sugars, and salt. Eat good food and let nature cure you of any disturbance to your natural systems

Lupus

Auto immune disease usually affecting women from teen years through 40's or 50's. African-Americans and native Americans are more often affected. 5 million cases worldwide and 16,000 new cases every year in America. Two main types of Lupus are discoid which mainly affects the skin and systemic which can affect internal organs, especially kidneys, and lead to cardiovascular disease which is the leading cause of death in long-term cases.

Symptoms. Extreme fatigue that doesn't go away with rest. Joint pain, and stiffness, in two or more joints. Fever over 100°F. Muscle pain. Hair loss. Skin sores and rashes (which may occur in a butterfly-shaped pattern across the cheeks and nose). Nose or mouth sores. Skin rashes after sun exposure.

Lupus is not contagious, not even through sexual contact. You cannot "catch" lupus from someone or "give" lupus to someone. Lupus is not like or related to cancer, however, some treatments for lupus may include immunosuppressant drugs that are also used in chemotherapy. Lupus can range from mild to life-threatening. With good medical care, most people with lupus can lead a full life.

Some people have an inherited predisposition to lupus and it may be triggered by something in their environment, and maybe some type of food. Avoid red meat. Eat foods rich in calcium. Avoid trans fats and processed foods. Try not to eat garlic and alfalfa. No salt. No alcohol.

Lupus is an inflammatory disease. So, it's possible, though not proven, that foods that fight inflammation could help lupus symptoms. On the other hand, foods that fuel inflammation could worsen them. Foods with possible anti-inflammatory properties include fruits and vegetables, which are rich in substances called antioxidants. In addition, foods containing omega-3 fatty acids, such as fish, nuts, ground flaxseed, canola oil, and olive oil may also help fight inflammation. It seems that possibly the disease is centered in white blood cells that give off an antibody that attacks skin and organs once they are stimulated by the genetics, but we don't know why

Lyme's Disease

Some black-legged deer ticks carry a small spirochete bacteria called Borrelia and can transfer it to a human in its bite. It is very difficult for our own immune system to find and kill the organism in our bodies because it changes its genetic markers and is able to hide in our blood and other tissues. It has a tail and can propel through the blood to all parts of the body including the brain.

Since Lyme disease is a multi-systemic illness there are a multitude of Lyme disease symptoms including: Flu-like illness, fever, history of tick bite (not all patients recall a bite), headache, extreme fatigue, rashes, deep red flush on cheek bones, red ear lobes, TMJ jaw pain, neck and back pain, joint pain and swelling, and bone pain. Sometimes the bite leaves a bulls-eye pattern on the skin.

But if it goes untreated, the infection can spread to the joints, the heart and the nervous system, which explains some of more advanced symptoms. Patients may suffer with severe headaches and neck aches, heart palpitations, facial palsy, and arthritis with severe joint pain.

The disease used to be confined to Long Island, New York, and Connecticut where it first was seen (it is named after the town of Old Lyme, Connecticut, where the original cases were diagnosed). Although incidence is still highest in the northeastern United

States, the disease has been reported throughout the country. You're at highest risk of encountering deer ticks in wooded areas, so be vigilant. When you're in infested areas, wear light colored clothing with long sleeves; be sure to tuck your pants into your socks to keep ticks from crawling up your legs. As soon as you get home, wash yourself and check your body for anything unusual. Have a partner check your back.

If you have good reason to believe you are infected, a couple of weeks of mild oral antibiotics can probably get rid of the bacteria if you get after it right away. The longer it hides and spreads in your body, the more difficult it is to totally eradicate. like any other disease, the better your health is when you are attacked, the better your chance of recovery. Can your immune system do the job without antibiotics? It is possible. Depends how bad is the infection and how good your immune system is. Some people can survive anything. They just have good health.

The bite often has many more organisms than Borrelia so the severity of the infection also depends on what they are and how much they all work together to affect your immune system. The multiple organisms can form slime deposits in your blood and are even more difficult for you to fight off. But it can be done.

Metabolic Syndrome

Metabolic syndrome is a cluster of conditions — high blood pressure, high blood sugar, excess body fat around the waist, and abnormal cholesterol or triglyceride levels. These often occur together, increasing your risk of heart disease, stroke, and diabetes. It means you can and should take some action before you are affected by those diseases.

Having just one of these conditions doesn't mean you have metabolic syndrome. However, having more than one of these might increase your risk even more.

If you have metabolic syndrome or any of its components, aggressive lifestyle changes can delay or even prevent the development of serious health problems.

Most of the disorders associated with metabolic syndrome have no symptoms, although a large waist circumference is a visible sign. If your blood sugar is very high, you might have signs and symptoms of diabetes — including increased thirst and urination, fatigue, and blurred vision.

At least 3 of the 5 following criteria must be met to diagnose a person with metabolic syndrome:

- Abdominal obesity: waist circumference of 40 inches in men and 36 inches in women
- Blood triglycerides over150 mg/dl
- Low HDL-Cholesterol under 40 mg/dL in men and under 50 mg/dL in women
- High blood pressure 130/85 mmHg
- High fasting glucose 110 mg/dl

Symptoms of metabolic syndrome:

Tiredness - particularly after meals

Inability to focus properly - brain fog

Acanthosis nigricans - browning of folds of skin such as on the neck, armpits, groin and between the buttocks

Abdominal obesity

Resistance to insulin

Migraine headache

The word migraine means half a head. That is the identifier of this type of headache. It settles on one side of the head. Not always, but usually. And the pain is intense. Throbbing. And there are visual disturbances, upset digestive tract, dizziness and extreme sensitivity to all your senses. 70% of migraine sufferers are female and actually can be any age, although the frequency and intensity seems to diminish with older age.

The headache tends to last for a few days and there is a recovery period of a day or two after the headache leaves. The person feels exhausted and just wants to sleep and maybe is a little unstable emotionally. What a relief that it is over, although some sufferers experience it more than once a month.

What causes the onset of the migraine? For some reason a person has brain blood vessels that go into spasm and constrict and then they relax and open wider than usual and some of your blood's fluid leaks out into that area of the brain. That doesn't cause the full-blown migraine but the fluid elicits and auto-immune response when your white blood cells cause your blood vessels to be damaged and inflamed and very sensitive. Then when the blood goes through normally, it can be very painful.

What causes the blood vessels to constrict and widen to begin with? With different people, naturally there are different factors such as excessive alcohol consumption, cigarette smoke, certain foods, exercise, normal fluctuations in our hormones, environmental factors and chemical imbalances. A brain chemical serotonin is also suspected of being often involved. Not eating enough foods containing magnesium night possible bring on an attack. Eat nuts, soybeans, green leafy vegetables, lemons, peaches, almonds, seeds, and whole grains might help. Of course, it is better to keep your magnesium levels high by eating good food before there is an attack.

Plenty of rest and sleep, cool compresses, and avoiding light and noise might help. Some alternative medical treatments that people use are acupuncture, chiropractic, and naprapathy. All those are directed keeping the blood flowing normally and relieving any blockages. No doubt, massage would also be beneficial. Probably the most important thing is to be eating good, natural foods and getting movement with your body.

Morgellon's Disease

"I have this weird, incurable disease that seems like it's from outer space. Morgellons is a slow, unpredictable killer — a terrorist disease: it will blow up one of your organs, leaving you in bed for a year. ... Fibers in a variety of colors protrude out of my skin like mushrooms after a rainstorm: they cannot be forensically identified as animal, vegetable or mineral." That is a description of Morgellon's disease from singer Joni Mitchell. She sometimes wouldn't wear clothing because she felt like she was being eaten alive — and that the disease left her confined to her house for several years.

Around 20,000 cases per year in the US. Symptoms generally include skin rashes, a sense of intense itching and crawling under the skin, and fatigue. The multi-colored filaments in the lesions of the disease are sort of a distinguishing characteristic. The fibers found in Morgellons skin lesions are not textile fibers, nor are they bugs or worms. They are human biofibers composed of the proteins collagen and keratin and produced by skin cells. While the blue coloration is caused by melanin pigmentation, the cause of red coloration is unknown.

Morgellons disease itself is not a mystery. A plausible explanation is supported by scientific evidence. The fibers are human structural proteins. It results from an aberrant response to the presence of tickborne pathogens. There is also the presence of brain lesions in some Morgellons patients. That confirms the non-delusional nature of the disease.

Symptoms of Morgellon's disease are: severe itching caused by sores or a rash, the feeling that insects are crawling under your skin, the feeling that you are being bitten or stung by insects, fibers or strings in or on your skin, the fibers may be in the sores, exhaustion, loss of concentration, memory loss, sleep problems, inflamed lymph nodes, abnormal reflexes, low body temperature.

Morgellons skin lesions are associated with Lyme disease and other tick-borne illnesses. To treat the skin condition one must first treat the underlying infection. Several laboratories have detected live Lyme bacteria directly in Morgellons skin tissue.

Bathe with a disinfectant, massage in olive oil, use a loofa to exfoliate the skin, eat a healthful diet with complex carbohydrates, whole grains, and green leafy vegetables. Nourishing vegetable juices and fresh fruits.

Mononucleosis (EBV)

This common and very contagious disease is caused by the Epstein-Barr Virus, EBV. 5 million people per year are carrying the virus. One common mode of transmission is through saliva and it is known as the kissing disease. Symptoms include fatigue, fever, rash, and swollen glands. The elderly may not have typical symptoms. Treatment involves rest, fluids, and over-the-counter pain and fever-reducing medicines to ease symptoms.

The EBV is a herpes virus and hides in our nervous systems for life. It can cause mono usually from kissing as teenagers. During later stressful times the virus reemerges and can cause long lasting symptoms of fatigue, flu-like symptoms and fever and it can last for a long time.

Women going through major life changes, including the death of a loved one, a major move or job change or menopause, for example, may be particularly susceptible to reactivation of the virus, and therefore a symptomatic infection. EBV reactivation can persist for months, Symptoms typically include fatigue, which can be quite intense, aching muscles and joints, swollen lymph nodes and other persistent flu-like symptoms. It can also cause malaise and even depression. A physical exam may find a swollen liver and spleen, and liver function tests may be abnormal.

Multiple Sclerosis (MS)

This is a truly devastating disease that affects people who seem to be in good, active health. More often, the disease strikes women. It is progressive and begins as a little discomfort and muscular weakness and sometimes the sufferer ends up in a wheelchair or even bedridden. It is an auto-immune disease in which your own white blood cells attack and destroy your Schwann Cells which surround the fibers on nerve cells and make an insulating myelin sheath around the fiber. Unfortunately, without the Myelin the nerve cells do not function properly, and the person starts to lose the use of the muscles that those nerve cells controlled.

How does this happen? Why do some people get it and others don't. For one thing, I believe they had bad luck. They have small genetic markers on the outer surface of the Schwann Cells that perfectly match genetic markers on the surface of a microorganism.

At the moment, we don't even know for sure what type of organism has the marker. A bacteria, a spirochete, a fungus, a virus. No one knows and no knows where the organism entered our body to cause an infection. In the colon or through the mouth. Sexually? We don't know. But it started an immune response with our white blood cells killing the invader. What our white cells do is multiply by the million, so they are ready if the invade comes back. They float in the bloodstream and find the marker on the Schwann Cells and begin to attack them. The beginning of MS.

Can anything be done? The Schwann Cells use oils to make the myelin. They need essential fatty acids (EFA's). They are essential because our body does not make them. We have to eat them. Linolenic acid and linoleic acid. Omega 3 and Omega 6. I think the best source for both of them is flaxseed oil. It is sort of expensive but, you don't need a lot of it. If your Schwann Cells are destroyed, they can't use the oil anyway, but I think you should provide the oil in case they are still functioning somewhat.

There are many new experimental therapies that are showing a lot of promise. Drugs to suppress the immune system from attacking the Schwann Cells, drugs to keep the white blood cells out of the brain area so they can't attack the myelin sheath, drugs to potentially rebuild the myelin. Eventually there will be a way for our body to identify and destroyed the white cells that are causing the MS. There are many hopeful cures in various stages of development. Some slow the disease progress and some retard the spread of the disease to other areas of your body. For now, I think massage and heat therapies are beneficial somewhat. It is a very difficult disease.

Osteoporosis

This is a disease of bone loss and can lead to breakage of bones especially on the femur at the hip, the bodies of the vertebrae (which leads to dowager's hump), and the wrist. Contributing factors are lack of calcium in the diet, lack of sunshine for the Vitamin D, and lack of exercise which adds to volume of bone mass. Women are more likely to have osteoporosis because for one thing, many of them had smaller bones since youth than men.

All of our bones are constantly being remodeled. We dissolve the old bone and make new bone. The process is sort of controlled by estrogen. As a person gets older the remodeling loses some of the rebuilding and bones get weaker.

Foods to avoid if you are in danger of osteoporosis.

Beans (Legumes)

While beans contain calcium, and magnesium, fiber and other nutrients, they are also high in substances called phytates. Phytates interfere with your body's ability to absorb the calcium that is contained in beans. You can reduce the phytate level by soaking beans in water for several hours and then cooking them in fresh water.

Salty Foods

Eating foods that have a lot of salt (sodium) causes your body to lose calcium and can lead to bone loss. Try to limit the amount of processed foods, canned foods and salt added to the foods you eat each day.

Spinach and Other Foods with Oxalates

Your body doesn't absorb calcium well from foods that are high in oxalates (oxalic acid) such as spinach. Other foods with oxalates are rhubarb, beet greens and certain beans. These foods contain other healthy nutrients, but they just shouldn't be counted as sources of calcium.

Wheat Bran

Like beans, wheat bran contains high levels of phytates which can prevent your body from absorbing calcium.

Alcohol

Drinking heavily can lead to bone loss. Limit alcohol to no more than 2 – 3 drinks per day.

Caffeine

Coffee, tea and soft drinks (sodas) contain caffeine, which may decrease calcium absorption and contribute to bone loss.

Coffee/Tea

Drinking more than three cups of coffee every day may interfere with calcium absorption and cause bone loss.

Soft Drinks

Some studies suggest that colas, but not other soft drinks, are associated with bone loss.

Some risk factors are out of your control, such as:

Gender

Osteoporosis is more common in women

Age

As you get older, your risk for osteoporosis increases

Body size

Small, thin women are at greater risk for osteoporosis

Ethnicity

White and Asian women have the highest risk for osteoporosis

Family history

If a biological family member has osteoporosis or breaks a bone, it's more likely that you will too

Calcium and vitamin D intake

You're more prone to bone loss if your diet is low in calcium and vitamin D

Medication use

Some medications may increase the risk of osteoporosis. Ask the doctor who prescribes your medications if this is the case

Activity level

Lack of exercise can weaken bones

Because Osteoporosis is silent, the bone density test, or DEXA, has become of major importance. The DEXA scan can tell you if your bone is becoming osteoporotic.

Fortunately, you can take steps to reduce your risk of osteoporosis. By doing so, you can avoid the often-disabling broken bones (fractures) that can result from this condition. If you already have osteoporosis, new medications are available to slow or even stop the bones from getting weaker. These medicines also can decrease the chance of having a fracture. I have been told that once you start these medications, you should never stop because your bones can then become weaker. But they do harden up the bones. I know a woman who was taking fosamax and fell down a flight of stairs and didn't break anything.

Parkinson's Disease

Usually the first symptom is tremors of the fingers, hand, and the chin. Especially at rest. There is no cure for the disease. There are certain cells in the brain that die and functioned to produce dopamine which is involved in movements. The medicines that are given for symptom relief are dopamine antagonists. They think the cause of the disease could be partially genetic and partially environmental, especially with exposure to toxins.

Another symptom of Parkinson's is difficulty with planning, initiating, and the execution of movements. Some people think they are moving so slow that they feel stiff. For example, they don't swing their arms when they walk, and they say they feel like their feet are nailed to the floor.

Some patients develop extreme rigidity in their movements because of excessive muscle contractions. And the contractions are not everywhere. For instance, the shoulders and neck muscled before the face and arm muscles. Another development in the disease is postural instability and can leads to falls and injuries and the patient loses self-confidence in their movements. The patient has difficulty beginning their walking and also difficulty stopping and may have to stop and turn to change direction. Their gait is often shuffling.

One of the early signs of Parkinson's is micrographia which is very small handwriting and not much spacing between words. There is also impaired recognition of facts, and time and also loss of ability for facial recognition. 78% of people with Parkinson's develop dementia and are 6 times more likely to develop dementia than the general population. The Parkinson's patient may develop hallucinations, paranoid fantasies, and delusions.

There is no known cure for Parkinson's, but there is hope for diminishing the symptoms and slowing the progression of the disease.

For natural therapy, the patient should be kept on a 100% raw food diet. Organically grown with emphasis on seeds, nuts ad grains. Especially sesame seeds and sesame butter. Sprouts, green leafy vegetables and juices. The key is a very low protein diet for Parkinson's.

Pneumonia

Pneumonia is an infection that inflames the air sacs in one or both lungs. The air sacs may fill with fluid or pus, causing cough with phlegm or pus, fever, chills, and difficulty breathing. A variety of organisms, including bacteria, viruses and fungi, can cause pneumonia. It is a big killer in hospitals and nursing facilities, often called iatrogenic pneumonia because the patient did not have the disease when they entered it.

The most common symptoms of pneumonia are: cough (with some pneumonias you may cough up greenish or yellow mucus, or even bloody mucus), fever, which may be mild or high, shaking chills, shortness of breath, which may only occur when you climb stairs.

Additional symptoms include: sharp or stabbing chest pain that gets worse when you breathe deeply or cough, headache, excessive sweating and clammy skin, loss of appetite, low energy, and fatigue. Confusion, especially in older people

Symptoms also can vary, depending on whether your pneumonia is bacterial or viral or fungal.

In bacterial pneumonia, your temperature may rise as high as 105 degrees F. This pneumonia can cause profuse sweating, and rapidly increased breathing and pulse rate. Lips and nail beds may have a bluish color due to lack of oxygen in the blood. A patient's mental state may be confused or delirious.

The initial symptoms of viral pneumonia are the same as influenza symptoms: fever, a dry cough, headache, muscle pain, and weakness. Within 12 to 36 hours, there is increasing breathlessness; the cough becomes worse and produces a small amount of mucus. There may be a high fever and there may be blueness of the lips.

Risk factors (increase your chances of getting pneumonia) :

Age younger than 5 and older than 65

Cigarette smoking

Recent viral respiratory infection—a cold, laryngitis, influenza, etc.

Difficulty swallowing (due to stroke, dementia, Parkinson's disease, or other neurological conditions), which can lead to aspiration (breathing in a foreign object)

Chronic lung disease such as COPD, bronchiectasis, or cystic fibrosis

Cerebral palsy

Other serious illnesses, such as heart disease, liver cirrhosis, or diabetes

Living in a nursing facility

Impaired consciousness (loss of brain function due to dementia, stroke, or other neurologic conditions)

Recent surgery or trauma

Some cases of pneumonia can be treated at home with the following measures:

Get as much rest as possible. If you have pneumonia, you need rest so that your body can fight the infection and heal. Don't try to do everything you normally do and rest when you feel tired. The more you're able to rest, the quicker you will get better.

Drink plenty of fluids. You hear this often no matter what illness you have, but it's really important. Drinking more water will help thin the mucus in your body, making it easier to expel when you cough, an important part of recovering from pneumonia. Drink broth, soup, tea, or even hot water to help ward off chills and get some extra hydration.

Drink a cup of caffeinated coffee or tea. Caffeine is known to be a mild bronchodilator and it's chemically similar to theophylline, a drug that's used to treat asthma. Studies have shown that caffeine can improve breathing by opening up the airways for up to four hours.

Take medications as directed. Your doctor may put you on an antibiotic, antiviral, or antifungal depending on what type of pneumonia you have. Make sure you take it as instructed and finish the entire prescription, even if you feel better.

Run a humidifier. Similar to drinking water, running a humidifier will keep your airways moist, especially when the air is dry in your house.

Gargle salt water. Gargling several times a day can help wash away some of the mucus in your throat and relieve a sore throat. If you hate salt water, gargling plain water works too.

Talk to your doctor about cough medicines. Because you need to cough to help get rid of the infection, talk to your doctor before taking any kind of a cough suppressant, even if your cough is making it difficult to sleep. You may be able to take a low dose of a cough medicine or your doctor might have other options.

Stop smoking and stay away from smoke. Smoke aggravates your symptoms and may prolong your recovery time.

Having a weakened immune system due to illness, certain medications, and autoimmune disorders.

Prostate

The prostate gland lies between the bladder and the urethra leading out of the body. It makes the seminal fluid that mixes with the sperm during ejaculation. Sometimes when men get older the prostate gland swells up in size and can possibly partially block the passage of urine from the bladder. There are two methods of surgery to open up the prostate. One is with a not electric needle and the other is with a laser to cut away some of the swollen glandular tissue. How do you know if you need help? There is a simple blood test that can indicate the amount of swelling in the prostate. Also a physician can reach through the anus and feel the prostate with is gloved finger. It is also the site for prostate cancer in men and he can pretty well determine if it is cancerous.

Psoriasis

Psoriasis is a chronic autoimmune condition that causes the rapid buildup of skin cells. This buildup of cells causes scaling on the skin's surface. Inflammation and redness around the scales is fairly common. Typical psoriatic scales are whitish-silver and develop in thick, red patches. Topical medicines to apply are: Salicylic acid . Some doctors recommend salicylic acid ointment, which smoothes the skin by promoting the shedding of psoriatic scales.

Steroid-based creams.

Calcitriol containing topical ointment.

Coal-tar ointments and shampoos.

Prescription retinoids

Even though these topical creams will give some temporary relief the condition at present is not curable.

Here are eight foods and beverages that get mentioned often by people as possibly causing their psoriasis flare-ups. You might consider cutting them out of your diet one at a time to see if any have an effect on your symptoms:

Alcohol First and foremost, stop drinking. Here's why: Alcohol opens the blood vessels in the skin. When your blood vessels are dilated, white blood cells, including the T cells that are believed to be responsible for psoriasis, can sneak into the outer layers of your skin more easily — and you don't need to be inviting more T cells. Your psoriasis symptoms may worsen even if you're a light to moderate alcohol user.

Junk Food Psoriasis is an inflammatory condition, and junk foods tend to be high in saturated and trans fats and refined starches and sugars, all of which can promote inflammation. Another reason to avoid junk foods is that that they are high in calories with little nutritional value, and people with psoriasis often have weight problems. If you have psoriasis, you have an increased risk of heart and vascular diseases. Being overweight adds to that risk.

Red Meat Red meats contain a polyunsaturated fat called arachidonic acid. This type of fat can worsen psoriasis symptoms because it can easily be converted into inflammatory compounds. Also to include on your foods-to-avoid list: processed meats, such as sausage and bacon.

Dairy Products Like red meat, dairy products also contain the natural inflammatory arachidonic acid. Cow's milk is one of the biggest culprits, because it also contains the protein casein, which has been linked to inflammation. Egg yolks, too, are high in arachidonic acid, so consider nixing them from your diet.

Nightshade Plants Some people report that consuming plants from the "nightshade fa — which includes peppers, white potatoes, eggplant, and tomatoes — exacerbates their psoriasis. These vegetables contain solanine, a chemical compound that has been shown to trigger pain in some people. Certain patients believe that if you avoid these vegetables, you decrease your symptoms.

Citrus Fruits Sometimes an allergic reaction can cause psoriasis to flare. Citrus fruits, such as grapefruit, oranges, lemons, and limes, are a common allergen. See if eliminating them from your diet improves your skin. This goes for their derivatives as well, such as lemonade and grapefruit juice.

Gluten This protein is found in some grass-related grains, including rye, wheat, and barley. Researchers in Portugal found that psoriasis symptoms in some people with a gluten sensitivity improved after they began avoiding gluten. Studies are ongoing, but the idea of psoriasis patients benefiting from a gluten-free diet is still controversial.

Condiments Some people with psoriasis find condiments and spices to be their enemy. The ones that seem to cause the most trouble for people with psoriasis are pimento, cinnamon, curry, vinegar, mayo, paprika, Tabasco sauce, Worcestershire sauce, and ketchup. These condiments are all on the no-no list because substances in each of them can increase inflammation.

Shingles

This very painful rash usually comes around the back towards the front of the torso. Heavy red rash with blisters that might open. Very sensitive and lasts for quite a while. Varicella is a herpes virus. It attacks many kids as chicken pox and then does the typical herpes routine of hiding, this one might hide near the spinal cord. Just like the genital herpes virus hides near the spinal cord and comes out along the path of a nerve when there is a flareup.

So what causes the flareup with shingles? Nobody knows yet for sure. Probably some kind of stress or environmental toxin. Or maybe something in your diet. Nobody knows. It just appears and stays for some weeks. One out of three people in the US have a case of shingles in their lifetime, but usually only one time, rarely several times. Analgesics (pain medicine) may help relieve the pain caused by shingles. Wet compresses, calamine lotion, and colloidal oatmeal baths may help relieve some of the itching.

Shingles cannot be passed from one person to another. However, the virus that causes shingles, the varicella zoster virus, can spread from a person with active shingles (in the blister phase) to cause chickenpox in someone who had never had chickenpox Once the rash has developed crusts, the person is no longer infectious.

Sjogren's Syndrome

This condition is not as rare as most people think. In the United States alone there are two million people afflicted, mostly women and often middle-aged, although children can be affected also. Like many other auto-immune diseases, the actual cause is unknown, and an actual cure is unknown. It usually does not get diagnosed right away because usually only a rheumatologist specialist can really diagnose it. Most patients

Dry mouth and dry eyes or just one of the places or possibly dryness in nasal passages, skin, and vaginal surfaces. Maybe swollen glands. It can lead to inflammation, pain and irritation. The physician involved will probably prescribe a medication used to treat the dryness, but it does not help the systemic disease of Sjogren's and the problems will return.

Is there anything that can be done to help the sufferer? At the moment our knowledge about auto-immune diseases is far from complete. We don't know the exact cause of Sjogren's although we do know what the pathological method of the disease is, but we can't really stop it. There are medications that help, but nothing that cures. We can suppress a person's immune system and give some relief during a flareup, but it will probably return again. Is it contagious? No. You either have it in your genes or you don't. Some microorganism probably starts the ball rolling when the person is exposed to it. We don't know what organism or how the exposure takes place. probably it is common, and many people are exposed to it, but you have to have some kind of genetic predisposition for it to cause Sjogren's. Someday we will know all about it. As for now, eat well and eat food that contain our natural immune suppressant, vitamin E, and keep yourself healthy.

Stomach Ulcers

Stomach and duodenal ulcers are usually due to one of two causes: the bacterium Helicobacter pylori or nonsteroidal anti — inflammatory drugs (NSAIDs) like aspirin, ibuprofen, and naproxen. An ulcer can cause abdominal pain, bleeding, or even cause a hole perforation. Both the H. pylori bacteria and the NSAID drugs have a tendency to degrade the mucus lining of the stomach that protects the inner walls from the peptic enzymes and acids which normally digest proteins in our food, but in this case they start to digest the walls of the stomach itself.

The bacterial cause of the ulcers was just discovered in the last 10 or 20 years when a scientist in Australia drank a bottle on television containing the H. pylori bacteria and soon he was examined with an endoscope and he was loaded with ulcers. The big benefit of his discovery was now doctors realize that ulcers must be treated with antibiotics. Previously they just medicated with antacids medications. Now they know there is a germ that must be killed.

It can be transferred person to person by sharing utensils or foods or liquids like water. Maybe from kissing. In some third world countries, entire villages get contaminated with the bacteria from deinking out of the same source, which may have been contaminated by feces from a infected person. Get rid of the bacteria and try to restore the stomach mucus. Also stop using the NSAID drugs.

Stroke

800,000 people per year suffer a stroke in America alone. It is the fifth biggest killer in this country and the number one cause of adult disability. There are two types of strokes. Hemorrhagic with too much blood spilling out into the brain, often from a broken aneurysm or damaged blood vessel. The second type is ischemic with not enough blood reaching a part of the brain because a vessel is possibly blocked by a blood clot. Wherever that vessel supplies blood to is where the damage will occur, possibly half the brain if the blockage is in one of the main arteries supplying the brain.

Some risk factors for having a stroke are not controllable. They just happen. Some risk factors can e improved. High blood pressure, artrial fibrillation rapid heartbeat and unusual feelings in the heart (AFib), high cholesterol, diabetes and circulation problems are all medical risk factors for stroke that A stroke is a medical emergency. Prompt treatment is crucial. Early action can minimize brain damage and potential complications.

The good news is that strokes can be treated and prevented, and many fewer Americans die of stroke now than in the past. Watch for these signs and symptoms if you think you or someone else may be having a stroke. Pay attention to when the signs and symptoms begin. The length of time they have been present can affect your treatment options.

Trouble with speaking and understanding. You may experience confusion. You may slur your words or have difficulty understanding speech. You may develop sudden numbness, weakness or paralysis in your face, arm or leg. This often happens just on one side of your body. Try to raise both your arms over your head at the same time. If one arm begins to fall, you may be having a stroke. Also, one side of your mouth may droop when you try to smile. Trouble with seeing in one or both eyes. You may suddenly have blurred or blackened vision in one or both eyes, or you may see double.

Headache. A sudden, severe headache, which may be accompanied by vomiting, dizziness or altered consciousness, may indicate you're having a stroke. Trouble with walking. You may stumble or experience sudden dizziness, loss of balance or loss of coordination. Seek immediate medical attention if you notice any signs or symptoms of a stroke, even if they seem to fluctuate or disappear. Think "FAST" and do the following:

Face. Ask the person to smile. Does one side of the face droop? Arms. Ask the person to raise both arms. Does one arm drift downward? Or is one arm unable to rise up? Speech. Ask the person to repeat a simple phrase. Is his or her speech slurred or strange? Time. If you observe any of these signs, call 911 immediately. Call your local emergency number right away. Don't wait to see if symptoms stop. Every minute counts, the greater the potential for brain damage and disability.

Trichomoniasis

Trichomoniasis is among the most common sexually transmitted infections. Risk factors include multiple sexual partners and not using condoms during sex. Trichomoniasis causes a foul-smelling vaginal discharge, genital itching, and painful urination in women. Many men typically have no symptoms. Some women also often have no symptoms. What is surprising is that a group with a high rate of infection is older women over the age of 50.

Complications include a risk of premature delivery for pregnant women. Trichomoniasis can also lead to inflammation of the vagina, urethra and cervix and to pelvic inflammatory disease. Treatment involves both partners taking one large dose of an oral antibiotic, usually metronidazole or tinidazole, which are effective in at least 95% of cases.

It is the most common curable STD in the United States with an estimated 3.7 million people infected. It is not common for the parasite to infect other body parts, like the hands, mouth, or anus, although sex toys can be a source of infection.

The parasite's name is Trichomonas vaginalis, also called Trich for short and is spread through sexual contact with an infected partner, either through penis-to-vagina intercourse or vulva-to-vulva contact. Signs of trichomoniasis may include a yellow-gray-green, frothy vaginal discharge with a foul or fishy odor. The vagina may be sore and red and may burn and itch. It may be painful to urinate or have sexual intercourse. However, many women with trichomoniasis do not have any symptoms. Vaginally applied medications may relieve the symptoms of trich, such as itching or swelling, but will not kill the parasite that causes the infection.

It is unclear why some people with the infection get symptoms while others do not. It probably depends on factors like a person's age and overall health. Infected people without symptoms can still pass the infection on to others. Having trichomoniasis can make it feel unpleasant to have sex. Without treatment, the infection can last for months or even years. People who have been treated for trichomoniasis can get it again. About 1 in 5 people get infected again within 3 months after receiving treatment. To avoid getting reinfected, make sure that all of your sex partners get treated. Also, wait 7-10 days after you and your partner have been treated to have sex again. Get checked again if your symptoms come back. Having trichomoniasis also makes it more likely for you to become infected with the HIV virus.

Varicose Veins

These are damaged veins most commonly seen just below the skin on the legs. Veins have a series of one-way valves that close after the heart beats so the blood doe not fall back towards the floor. So the heart beats and the valves close so the blood is kept moving back towards the heart. If the valve is damaged, then the blood sort of pools in the veins and forms the varicosity. Hemmorhoids are an example of varicose veins besides on the legs.

Some people claim that ye ultimate cause of varicose veins is sitting too much and not getting enough exercise, like walking or swimming. Get plenty of

Vitamin C and the foods and juices associated with it. White oak bark tea ad witch hazel, Exercise on a slant board with your head downward. Elastic stockings to push some of that excess blood into the deeper veins. Avoid constipation by eating food with fibers

Vertigo

A spinning sensation or dizziness is the most frequent reason older folks seek medical help. It can lead to falling and is quite dangerous. Falling is a common cause of death among older people. Vertigo itself is usually related to the inner ear where we have organs of balance. There can be inflammation or an infection or small particles formed in the inner ear.

Here is a home remedy that a person can do on their own:

For dizziness from the left ear and side:

1. Sit on the edge of your bed. Turn your head 45 degrees to the right.

2. Quickly lie down on your left side. Stay there for 30 seconds.

3. Quickly move to lie down on the opposite end of your bed. ...

4.   Return slowly to sitting and wait a few minutes.

5.   Reverse these moves for the right ear.

If you tend to experience repeated episodes of dizziness, consider these tips:

Be aware of the possibility of losing your balance, which can lead to falling and serious injury.

Avoid moving suddenly and walk with a cane for stability, if needed.

Fall-proof your home by removing tripping hazards such as area rugs and exposed electrical cords. Use nonslip mats on your bath and shower floors. Use good lighting.

Sit or lie down immediately when you feel dizzy. Lie still with your eyes closed in a darkened room if you're experiencing a severe episode of vertigo.

Avoid driving a car or operating heavy machinery if you experience frequent dizziness without warning.

Avoid using caffeine, alcohol, salt and tobacco. Excessive use of these substances can worsen your signs and symptoms.

Drink enough fluids, eat a healthy diet, get enough sleep and avoid stress.

If your dizziness is caused by a medication, talk with your doctor about discontinuing it or lowering the dose.

If your dizziness comes with nausea, try an over-the-counter (nonprescription) antihistamine, such as meclizine or dimenhydrinate (Dramamine). These may cause drowsiness. Nondrowsy antihistamines aren't as effective. If your dizziness is caused by overheating or dehydration, rest in a cool place and drink water or a sports drink (Gatorade, Powerade, others).

Epley maneuver carried out by a doctor: this is designed to reposition crystals that have formed in the inner ear and contributing to the person's vertigo.

Ask the person to sit upright on an examination table, fully extending their legs out in front of them.

Rotate the person's head at a 45-degree angle towards the side they are experiencing the worst vertigo.

Quickly push the person back, so that they are lying down with their shoulders touching the table. The person's head is kept facing the side worst affected by vertigo but now at a 30-degree angle, so that it is lifted slightly off the table. The doctor holds the person in this position for between 30 seconds and 2 minutes, until their dizziness stops.

Rotate the person's head 90 degrees in the opposite direction, stopping when the opposite ear is 30 degrees away from the table. Again, the doctor holds the person in this position for between 30 seconds and 2 minutes, until their dizziness stops.

Next, they roll the person in the same direction that they are facing, onto their side. The side that they experience the worst vertigo on will be facing upwards. The doctor holds the person in this position for between 30 seconds and 2 minutes, until their dizziness stops.

Finally, the doctor brings the person back up to a sitting position.

The whole process is repeated up to three times, until the person's symptoms are relieved.

Vaping

When you smoke a tobacco cigarette you will be inhaling over 7,000 chemicals in the tobacco and paper. Many of those have to be toxic and certainly contribute to the condemnation that cigarettes are given. They are a hazard to your health if you smoke them on a regular basis.

There has been lots of publicity about cigarettes and lots of kids are scared of smoking tobacco cigarettes because of the health dangers. But they are not scared of smoking e-cigarettes. It is not exactly smoking. It is properly called vaping. Most teenagers have tried vaping and many of them get their first experience with nicotine by vaping. Teenage addiction rates to nicotine are high. Nicotine is one of the most physically addicting substance known to humankind. The kids are hooked, and it is legal. At some schools the kids stand around in the bathroom vaping, so there is social pressure to join in and the addiction is strong and widely shared.

Th e e-cigarette has a battery-operated heating coil called an atomizer and the user adds a capsule with nicotine and flavorings. A mist or vapor is formed as the user inhales it. There is not really any smoke because the mixture is not being burned. It is just vaporized. It seems to be more socially acceptable among younger users. They all like the feeling of the nicotine scrambling up their brains, but now most of them do not condone tobacco use and tobacco is not allowed in schools and restaurants and many homes. Many parents think the vaping is acceptable. Addicting, but acceptable.

The younger they start the more severe can be the addiction. People end up in counselling. Even in substance abuse facilities and their only substance is the nicotine. Many cases of anxiety. Inability to concentrate. Learning disorders. Attention deficit. The brain circuits underlying pleasure and the pursuit of enjoyable experiences develop much faster than the circuits that promote decision making, impulse control and rational thinking.

It is not just kids who do vaping. A lot of older adults who are trying to ease off tobacco use the vaporizers for their nicotine fix, but they do prefer the smoke going into their lungs and the stimulation from the vaping is not as satisfying to regular tobacco users. The e-cigarettes are not FDA approved as tobacco cessation devices, like patches and gum.

In many countries e-cigarettes are illegal, but here in the US, the e-cigarettes are legal and becoming more and more socially acceptable and popular. Especially with young people. It is a legal high. Ok at school or on a job. You probably won't get so high that you will be noticed or criticized. It is an easy addiction and really not overly expensive. Probably about the same cost or a little less than regular cigarettes. But it is an addiction. Nicotine addiction. And there can be withdrawal symptoms and cravings. And there may be more ingredients in the vapor than is advertised, so the possibility of toxicity does exist.

Chapter 4

Dr. Cargill's Notebook

In the beginning

Exactly when is the beginning of a new person's life is really unknown. A lot of theories, but nobody knows anything for sure. Especially when it comes to the spiritual aspects of that new person being formed. Like for instance, there are possibly memories from before the baby is even developing in the womb. Nobody knows how it works, but the child is born with behavioral characteristics and awareness somehow attributable to the parents. So, more is passed during fertilization that just genes for physical development. The sperm and the egg are alive and possess an amount of the person's spirit. Is it a lot? Who knows? We don't understand the spirit yet.

DNA is a very complex chemical used in passing genetic information from one generation to the next through the sperm and egg. I personally became convinced there is a God after I studied DNA structure. It is way too complicated to have just happened by itself.

I believe carbohydrates, lipids, and proteins could just develop naturally in nature, maybe along a seashore and with powerful sunshine. Who knows? Scientists have created those chemicals naturally in labs. But that does not make them alive. To be alive would probably require some kind of reproduction and that would require some DNA, which would never form just in nature. So, what I am saying is that life could never just form by itself. It has to be created.

So anyway, the baby develops inside the mother and then is born. It has been deriving its nourishment from the mother's blood. Her blood is replenished from her food intake and possibly by "cannibalizing" her own tissues if necessary. After the child is born, it will be preferably fed on his mother's own milk. It seems like that would be the best next step because her milk is perfectly suited for her child, and also the child would develop i's own immune system from the mother.

I am going to provide here a very simplified description of the human immune system. Being exposed to bacteria and viruses causes activation of white blood cells in our blood stream, including in a baby. Some of these white blood cells ingest germs and kill them and others excrete our chemical and protein defenses called antibodies. Those stick to the invading bacteria or virus and signal for the white blood cells that eat germs to get busy.

The developing baby starts to develop some of the immune system defenses from the placenta in the last few months of pregnancy and also when the baby is exposed to bacteria, yeasts, and viruses coming through the birth canal. This exposure causes the baby's immature immune system to start making antibodies that will protect it throughout its life. Of course, in a C-section the baby does not get exposed to those organisms at birth. So the immune system is somewhat compromised in C-section births.

Nature provides another source for the little baby to get some antibody protection, mother's breast milk and colostrum, an early milk. These are made in the breast by organs that make milk by extracting nutrients from the mother's blood and also bring along some of her antibodies that the baby uses for its immune system. Her antibodies multiply in the baby's blood, and the baby "remembers" the protection for life.

Natural birth, natural breast feeding, and maybe the most important is the mother eating natural foods during the pregnancy. Full of all the proper nutrients so her child can have a fair chance to develop into a healthy person. All the little cells in the developing baby are dividing and growing. You want them to do it perfectly and rapidly. Nothing missing. There is a program for development. It is natural in every pregnancy. You want it to be perfect in the plan. If there is something different then the results can only be negative. You can't make the child better than natural. Any changes will be negative.

A mother should definitely not want to put any substances into her body that are not natural. Natural is where it's at. Natural is the peak. It is your child. Carrying your genes and your family's genes for a thousand years. If you abuse your genes, they cannot be restored. Let your genes flourish and create a wonderful person. The key word is natural. It doesn't get any better than natural.

Probably the majority of Americans, maybe the majority of people in the world, feed their children some kind of milk after they are too old for nursing to be necessary. It is not necessary. Maybe it is done for convenience. Maybe because it is a tradition. Maybe milk for a child is satisfying to a deep psychological need. Maybe they feel the child is better assured of getting all of its nutritional needs. But that is not necessary if the parents will make an effort to carefully prepare the child's food from non-milk sources. Vegetable sources can be adequately nutritious to properly feed the child.

It is important that the child's colon is replete with probiotic lactobacilli that are our friendly bacteria able to help defend the child from invasion by pathogenic microorganisms. Well, the child should already have those probiotic helpers from his mother's placenta and later from her breast milk. Yes, it is important to breast feed. Especially the colostrum at the beginning. It is loaded with helpers for the child's system. Those health promoting ingredients are not found in any formula. Absolutely none.

Holism

What is holism? It is a mysterious term. Almost mystical. I have no idea who originated the term, but over the years it has been reinterpreted many times. A lot of additions to it. Attempts at streamlining it. Almost any discipline now can have holistic aspects. It's an in thing.

No factor should be considered without it's full complement of associated factors. Nothing is isolated. Everything is a part of a whole. Maybe more than one whole. I am a physician, so I am using the concept of holism to apply to the health of a human being. Does that also include other life forms like animals and plants? Yes, it does. The scientific concepts are the same for all life. The actual applications of those concepts vary from species to species.

My personal concentration is with humans. And there are no differences among humans. Everyone is the same. Maybe a little more of this or a little less of that among individuals, but there is absolutely nothing that can be measured to classify a person into a particular group.

A holistic physician is someone who attempts to consider all aspects of his patients. He doesn't look for a specific particular cause of a problem and naturally does not treat that particular cause specifically. All aspects of a patient must be considered. It is impossible to determine an exact cause without considering the whole person.

Often the triad of holistic health is body, mind, and spirit. That's a good start. It would seem to be all-encompassing and anything else that affects a patient's well-being can probably be fit into one of those general categories.

As for actual treatment in a holistic manner, it is not the usual way things are done. Most practitioners have a hard-enough time just effecting one of those aspects of their patient. Maybe in a really beneficial setting, the patient should be seen by a team of therapists who each are especially adept at working on a particular aspect of a patient's situation.

The benefit of being treated holistically is that the practitioner will not just latch onto a symptom and just do something to alleviate it. For instance, if the patient has a pain and the practitioner provides a medicine to relieve the pain. Certainly, that can be an amazing relief, but usually that does not relieve the cause of the pain and very likely the pain will return when the medicine "wears off".

Most physicians today have at least a holistic attitude somewhat. They know there is an underlying cause or causes to the pain or malfunction. The problem is the load of patients waiting for the physician's time, so the physician tries to provide some fast relief to a patient's discomfort instead of trying to find out the underlying cause of it.

The underlying cause is probably very complicated by a series of factors that have been building up for a while. The physician usually tries to pass the patient on to a type of specialist to do a part in untangling the web of symptoms. And that specialist really only knows their particular technique or specialty and that patient's underlying disorder has probably still not been considered.

I call it production-line health. There are not enough practitioners for the many, many sick people. So the doctors try to keep their patient's alive and reasonably comfortable. That is all they have time to do. They often have thousands of patients. They can only give you say half an hour a year or less. Even if they like you.

Your underlying causes still have not really been addressed by the medications and probably you will eventually be lined up for some kind of surgery or heavier therapy, more temporary alleviation and possibly leading to complications and worsening of your condition and after-effects. Your underlying condition now might be even more difficult to treat effectively.

Is there any hope? Can you ever get off the health production line? Obviously, it is best to never get on it. Develop and maintain bountiful health for life naturally. I believe if your body is strong and properly functioning that your mind and spirit will also be benefitted. There will of course, be some deterioration and also accidents leading to lessening of your powers and that makes it a lot more difficult to maintain good health. And many people imbibe substances that are detrimental to their health.

So what I am saying is that if you maintain good physical health, the rest will fall into place. The two main activities that you can do to promote your health are proper eating and proper movements and care of your physical structure. Your body, mind, and spirit are part of the whole. They make you who you are. In this book, I will discuss ways for you to be forever healthy. No medicines, no surgeries, no psychotherapy. The key is the word natural.

Evolution of Love

All land animals have sex with the male behind the female, except for humans. Scientists think that ape females have instant orgasms, but when humans started having intercourse from the front, the females did not orgasm as easily and lost their reward for allowing the male to enter them. The female pre-humans had large teeth and could be very threatening to the males who wanted to have sex. It was a crisis in our development because without sex the species would die out.

Some smarter males figured out what females do like; cuteness as in the young, so the males tried to act cute, also some security so the males began to provide some food and security for the females, and friendship, so the males started becoming friends with the females. Those three factors, cuteness, security, and friendship led to the development of love between them and both sexes were happy.

Tau Ma Tincture of Marijuana

I had studied Chinese herbal medicine and one of their drugs was called Tau Ma, which means "The Mother" and they used it for a variety of maladies. I prepared it by soaking marijuana stems and some leaves and buds in pure grain alcohol and the result was a bright iridescent green tincture. It had to be stored in dark glass because light going through clear glass would cause rapid deterioration.

According to the doctrine of signatures in herbal medicine, if a medicine was negatively affected by light it should be effective against fungi which thrive in the dark. I used it several times in cases of severe external fungal infection and it was the only thing that was effective. A friend had been bitten by a fish and an infection was spreading over his hand. It looked terrible. The Tau Ma cleared it up. The Chinese also used it against any type of internal infection.

My mother was bedridden sick for about a week and I felt she might die and she didn't want to see a medical doctor. I convinced her to drink some Tau Ma in an herbal tea and the next day she got up began cleaning house. It worked.

Muscle Cramps

Usually related to a dietary deficiency or the inability of your body to assimilate the nutrients from your diet. Symptoms are usually aggravated at night or when you are inactive. Deficiencies particularly magnesium, calcium, potassium, vitamin B6 and vitamin D. A heat pack and massage may help. Foods to eat: leafy green veggies, apricots, fruits, millet, sesame seeds, almonds. Avoid excess citrus, excess wheat, avoid all meat. Try carrot juice, beet juice, cucumber juice. Dandelion tea and alfalfa tea.

Pineal gland

Ancient people called it the third eye. It does have sensory fibers attached to the optic nerve and it measure the amount of light that we take in. Why is this important? When we were primitive and living more in nature, our sexual activity was controlled by the light sensors. We would want, our children born in spring or early summer so they would have a better chance of survival, so if you count back 9 months it is the fall and even today our sexual activity peaks then which is when the days get shorter, so less light to the pineal and more sex hormones produced.

William McDonagh DO

Conventional medicine treats patients after the establishment of disease. Early detection and prevention is ignored. Usually irreversible structural change follows functional change that has been in progress for months or years. When "modern medicine" states "nothing abnormal found" but the patient has obvious complaints, the sufferer must wait until he can exhibit sufficient, unmistakable morbidity to be eligible for treatment. At this point the system cranks up to do battle with a vast array of expensive drugs, specialist physicians, surgeries, and hospitalization time. Advanced degenerative diseases are rarely reversed or cured but controlled so long as the patient continues under the care of his or her physician.

Naprapathy

Medicine is the science and practice of the diagnosis, treatment, and prevention of disease. Naprapathy (na prah' pathy) is a system of medicine based upon keeping all our joints healthy which means unimpeded in our movements and pain free. Healthy joints probably will result in general good health, provided the person does not abuse themselves with poor nutrition and other obvious detriments to good health. Naprapathy especially concentrates on the spine to make sure every part of the body gets proper nerve stimulation

Rolling Thunder

Most medicine men have their own peculiar methods and equipment, and it's considered a matter of pride that each one works out an individual routine and doesn't copy anyone else. Of course, a new healer can watch another's procedure and get some idea of what to do, but the novice gradually develops the substance of a personal ritual, including the songs, prayers, and chants that are used.

Here are a few general guidelines from Rolling Thunder, a native medicine man, that can apply to the methods of almost all native healers. In the first place, it's best to conduct healing rituals in a natural setting, in the open air. My home is where I live and rest. I don't want negative forces hanging around.

Second, I never charge anything for healing. It's said, among our people, that if a medicine man sells his services or commercializes his ability in any way, he'll lose his power. Third, I don't make any guarantees for my cures, either, simply because nothing is absolutely sure in this life. Fourth, if a person comes to me with an open mind and an open heart, chances are good we can find the answer to his or her problem.

Juices and herbs for liver cleansing

Do you have indications of liver problems? Elevated liver enzymes in your blood test? Swelling under the bottom of your right rib cage? Clay colored stools? Dark urine? Try these fresh juices: red beet juice from tops and roots, lemon juice, papaya juice, grape, radish, dandelion juices added to the beet juice.

Herbs: dandelion, horsetail, St. John's wort, lobelia, sarsaparilla, golden rod, parsley

Kidney disease

The kidneys are composed of millions of tiny urea filters called nephrons. Kidney disease means damage to the nephrons. High blood pressure can cause it. Also if the urine backs up into the kidneys because the prostate is blocked. Probably you will not regrow new nephrons so the important thing is to protect the ones you have left. How do you know the condition of your kidneys? A blood test measuring the creatinine levels and blood urea nitrogen levels is one way. Urinalysis also can tell if your blood proteins are leaking out. Reduce your blood pressure and eat more fresh vegetable and less concentrated protein because that is where the urea comes from.

Fruitarian

When I was a young guy coming up, I remember reading about fruitarians and there was one guy, Ted PanDeva Zagar, over in East Chicago, Indiana working at the library and he hosted vegan potlucks there and I was honored to speak at one of them. A fruitarian does not kill anything. Not animal and not plants.

They eat plants as long as the plant is not killed in the process, for instance, leaf lettuce. The stricter California fruitarians also would not eat any part of a plant if it interfered with the plant's reproductive cycle. Very spiritual people.

Dr. Arnold Ehret

Fruit is the only cuisine that is karmaless. All other food involves killing whether it be of animals, plants, or seed. When ripened to perfect by the sun, it is plucked from the tree by the wind and laid as an offering for human kind or animals. It is the easiest food to digest. It is the least mucus forming of all foods.

Dr. Paavo Airola: Cause of disease

According to my hero, Dr. Paavo Airola, all diseases have the same underlying cause, prolonged physical and mental stresses, such as faulty nutritional patterns, constant overeating, overindulgence in proteins, severe emotional stresses, nutritional deficiencies, sluggish elimination of toxins, lack of exercise, and lack of relaxation. Bacteria and viruses are more often the result of disease rather than the cause.

Calcium

Everyone knows we need it for strong bones and teeth, but it is used in all bodily processes, sort of as an electrolyte to make things work. Besides osteoporosis, deficiency in calcium can cause nervousness, depression, insomnia, and irritability. Good natural sources include dark green leafy veggies, sesame and sunflower seeds, millet, walnuts, oats, navy beans, tortillas. Of course, it doesn't get absorbed unless you have some Vitamin D, of which the best source is sunshine on your skin.

Mental conversions

I've been reading about other unusual stuff like a lot of people in the same town coming up with the same jerky motions and stuttering like it was a contagious disease. One person to another. Starts in the mind and is expressed in their bodies. another thing I read is when two people meet who really like each other, their feet tap the same number of times. Some kind of mental transference between them and then expressed in their fee

Maya Angelou To love ourselves

One of our greatest challenges is learning to love ourselves, then having the courage and the wisdom to love others. We don't know how or why love occurs. Love is one of the most important emotions and is an instrumental key to unlocking the inner doors of our ignorance and fear.

OPTOSIS suicide of the mind. Swedish Resignation Syndrome

There is an epidemic of this strange condition in Sweden right now. Hundreds of children have started losing interest in life and then shut down the conscious part of their brain. Their brain stem keeps the child alive as long as the parents feed them with tubes. Physically, there's nothing wrong with them. They have lost the will to live. The condition is thought only to exist in Sweden. The children affected by the condition start showing symptoms by withdrawing from social activities and speaking less, before finally closing off completely from the world around them. They become a Sleeping Beauty. It also happened in Jamestown in 1610. About 50 healthy young men died from optosis. When their ship finally returned after a year, they were all dead and no violence. Just lost the will to live. and they did have adequate food and water

Two women can have a child

When I was at the University everything I wanted to do will be done 50 years from now. I was 50 years ahead of my time and administrators were only concerned about grant money. For instance, I had it all worked out technically how I could use the DNA from two women so they could have a child together and both be the biological parents. And I was working on doing the same for two men.

Women and sex

Women have more to lose. For one thing she might get pregnant and that is a biggie. She might get an STD. There are a lot of them and guys are slick at removing condoms without you even knowing it. What about emotions? Guys are sensitive also, but the archetypal image is a woman seduced and abandoned. The dude moves on down the line and she suffers sometimes for years. It can work the other way also, but not usually, because guys forget pretty quickly when they are on to something new. Women seem to put more of their heart into lovemaking, but not always. Who knows. It is a chance you take.

Female and male sexuality

Many females really do not want to have sex with someone unless she cares for that person. Loves. A male wants to do it anyway and the love develops in the process. Where is the middle ground? That is the age-old question. So hard to break the ice.

Fasting against cancer

Cachexia is the body's last-ditch weapon against cancer. If it doesn't work, then the patient will probably die. Cachexia is a self-induced state of starvation and when this happens, the blood chemistry remains normal by digesting proteins in the body's tissues. The first things to go will be abnormal growths, i.e. tumors and other cancer-caused structures, even cancerous cells. Fasting has this same effect. Do it for a week once a year to nip little growths in the bud.

Happiness

How do you know if you are happy? Do you chuckle to yourself? Do you think about enjoyable times? Do you smile at people? Total strangers? Do you care that someone else is made happier by your cheerfulness? Are you patient? Setbacks are accepted not dwelled upon. Are you optimistic that things will get better? Do it. Get it done. With a song in your voice when you talk. Or when you write to someone. Be glad you are alive. Enjoy doing whatever you do. If you believe in God, then praise God. You are healthy and strong and happy.

Cure for a sore muscle

Let's say the left biceps hurts when you lift your hand towards your shoulder. Could be some fibers torn or kind of stuck together. Face the palm towards the shoulder. Bring the hand towards the shoulder. Place your right hand on your left forearm. Now start stretching the left arm open. Then stop and try to bring it up again, but this time resist with your right hand. Do it hard. Then stretch more. Repeat it a few times each time stretching more until the arm is all the way open and your left bicep is back to normal. This works with any muscle in the body. Even small face muscles that need to be stretched and strengthened. Contract and then stretch.

Flatulence

The enzyme in saliva is called salivary amylase. It breaks chains of carbohydrates called complex carbs into more manageable small groupings.

That's important because your stomach's digestive juices are mainly concerned with proteins. If you didn't chew thoroughly and mix your food with saliva, then the complex carbs will enter the intestines as complex carbs and may not get digested at all because the small intestine's enzymes need simple carbs to function, not complex.

And they probably will go into the colon as complex carbs. There they will be acted upon by the natural bacterial flora in your colon. The by-product is gas, methane, intestinal gas. Chew your food well or you will be flatulent.

Eat for Health

It all comes down to what you eat. There are other factors, of course, like the air you breathe and the water you drink, that may have a big effect on your health. And how about our mental attitude towards things? Do happier people live longer? I don't know that a study has ever been done relating attitude to longevity. And how could you tell if someone has been a happier person. And anyway, if you are not happy, there is probably not much you can do about it. It is you.

But our food intake is something we do have control over. For one thing, smaller particles are easier to digest and absorb, hence the value of soup. Chew your food until you can drink it. Don't swallow big stuff. Too hard for your body to break it down. Even if it is a mushy type of food, still chew it. Your saliva begins the process of digestion. Complex carbs into simple carbs.

Colonic irrigation

Patient lies on his side and is covered. a unit is inserted into rectum painlessly. it has 2 tubes, one bringing fresh water in and the other coming out for material from your colon that leads to a sewer line. There is a sight glass so the therapist can see what is coming out. "Oh, a nice chunk." Feels wonderful. Especially when they clean out the cecum with accumulated toxins. The cecum is kind of a dead end at the furthest point from your rectum. Stuff can lay in there for years if it is not cleaned out.

Large Butts

Researchers at the Oxford University have released the results of a research that suggests that women who had bigger behinds had lower risks of coming down with diseases. It also went on to say that such women turned out to be smarter than their counterparts.

Everything points to the fact that women with smaller waists, wider hips and bigger butts have the longer life expectancies when compared to other women.

Eat to defecate

Constipation can be controlled by eating natural food with fiber. It tickles the walls of the intestines and the muscles contract and pushes the feces along. There is no fiber in meat or dairy or white flour and not much in potatoes without the skins. You gotta think this every meal. Every bite. Think about if the wastes are going to be moving out naturally or clogging up. Sometimes there is there is so much impacted fecal matter caused by constipation that there is just a small opening in the colon to barely squeeze anything out. I have been told by a colon therapist that she removed twenty pounds of impacted fecal matter from one person. The cause is not enough fiber. If you are chronically constipated, see a colon therapist for an irrigation procedure. It feels wonderful to be really cleaned. Prices vary. Somewhere between 50 and a hundred dollars. Then start over, now with a more healthful diet.

Colon cancer

I hear so much about colon cancer. I knew a few people personally who died of it in the past two years. The colon is kind of a mysterious area. We are aware of it, but we can't see it and hopefully, we don't feel it. In my opinion the best way to prevent colon cancer is to keep the feces moving out of it.

Does constipation cause colon cancer? No one knows for sure, but it makes sense that the health of the colon is better if it is functioning normally and emptied thoroughly and regularly. How does a person ensure that? Eating natural fiber-containing foods.

Peristalsis is waves of muscle contractions through the digestive system that pushes the material that we ate along and when enough is ready, it is expelled in a bowel movement. Peristalsis is created when fiber touches the intestinal walls. It causes the muscles to contract.

There is no fiber in meat or dairy products or eggs. Also in most highly processed foods, the fiber is removed or destroyed. Eat whole grains, fresh fruits and vegetables, brown rice, beans, nuts. A hamburger on a white bun has almost no fiber. The food moves very slowly through your system and is there for several days instead of I day which is normal for food with fiber.

Since it lays around inside you for a long time, then any toxins or chemicals in the meat or food will have a longer time to be absorbed into the walls of the colon. I believe constipation is often a contributing cause of colon cancer.

Food Bills

Dear Dr. Cargill, I am your facebook friend and I would like your opinion. My food bills add up to $500 every month. Does that sound like a lot for one woman? Sophie

Dear Sophie. I hope I am not being too coarse, but I think you are either overweight or you waste a lot of food. You didn't specify if you were eating out a lot.

That is a whole different situation. I am assuming the $500 is your grocery bills and really to me that seems like a lot. And I eat good food. I think a single person eating well should be able to get by on $400 a month or maybe even less.

A Woman

I want a real woman Not one just growing up. I don't care about your age or whether you are beautiful. I would prefer that you aren't beautiful. although I really like a shapely hip area. I would like you to have yourself together enough that you don't have to be concerned about my lifestyle. And my beliefs are good. Equality of all people. No abusing animals. Preservation of the Earth. The right to peacefully protest anything. There is a God creator who put it all together. It didn't just happen. I can talk with you on almost any subject. I am not looking to change you and vice-versa.

Margarine

I ate a lot of margarine growing up. My parents would never have given anything to their kids if they thought it was harmful, but they fell for all the advertising praising this miracle healthy butter substitute. It is made by pumping hydrogen into various vegetable oils to make it hard like butter and it is called hydrogenated. It is artificial, a synthetic. Our body uses it to make the cell walls of every cell in our body. Luckily, I learned many years ago about the danger of artificial hydrogenated oils and I stopped eating it long ago. After 7 years, all our cells have been replaced. By the way read the labels on the peanut butter you feed your kids. is it hydrogenated oil, salt, sugar, and peanut flavoring? Throw it in the garbage and get real peanut butter made of real peanuts. Just ground up peanuts. That's all.

Sugar Addiction

Dear Dr. Cargill; I'm addicted to sugar. Do you have any suggestions on how to break that addiction.? Rita W.

Dr. Cargill: I don't think sugar is actually physically addicting so it just takes will power and determination to stop. How about not having any sugar items in your home? I've seen claims that sugar cravings may be related to nutritional deficiencies or some kind of psychological distress, genetic predisposition, or past alcoholism.. Many, many explanations, but none of them verifiable. Don't bring sugary items home or eat and drink sugar at a location. Stay away from places that feed your craving for their profit. Your will power is based on your self-esteem. If sugar is destroying your body and personality, you have to rise above it and realize your personal worth. Just do it. Stop right now. Get rid of it now. Try it Rita. You have no physical addiction like cocaine or heroin. You just have to really want to quit and then quit. Now. You are worth it.

Human Cloning

Can human cloning be done? Yes, easily. I was on a team that cloned mice and rats and sheep. Humans can be done, but it is illegal because our lawmakers really don't understand the technology and the implications of the science. I am sure it is being done right now in secret labs. It is easy to remove the DNA that controls the creation of the cerebrum part of the brain and leave the brain stem intact and that controls heart beat and breathing so the clone would be left alive and fed through tubes for many years, but in a coma. Why Is it being done? Spare parts for the super-rich. A perfect match for transplants if they need anything. A lot of precise work in making the fertilized egg for a clone. After that, anyone can implant the embryo into a surrogate and feed and care for the clone. Not many people know how to make the fertilized egg for a clone that will be kept alive in a coma.

Selling your eggs

Many college women pay part of their tuition by selling some of their eggs to fertility clinics to be used for helping women with defective eggs get pregnant. The donor's nuclear DNA will be removed from the egg, however there will still be mitochondrial DNA left so some of the donor's genes will be passed to the new baby. The donor will be given hormones to get her to release probably several hundred eggs which are gathered by the clinic. You have several million eggs so there will not be a serious depletion of your own childbearing ability and it pays well.

Steam Room

Just returned from a health club, shower, steam, whirlpool, swimming pool and a shave. I feel great. Some doctor friends don't think steam is the answer, but I like cleaning out my pores. Sweat glands are like miniature kidneys. and I lost a couple pounds.

Gut feelings

Go with them. I think it is some kind of inner spirit protection that is our life force trying to stay alive. Or maybe a guidance from a guardian angel. I am a scientist. Always have been and that is my Mensa category, but I really believe in going with a gut feeling. Some kind of protective shield for us. You just know something is bad for you and it probably is.

Polish Inn

I was shocked by the super obesity of the patrons there. Not just normal overweight Americans, but people who are disabled by their obesity. It is a good buffet dinner, but people sit and eat and sit and eat and sit and eat. And some of them probably go there every day. I like some of the food, but I can't go there any more after seeing those people. The place was packed with them. Scared me off.

Defecation

According to a recent American Mensa Journal, defecation is something that will be eliminated by producing super-efficient foods that have very little waste left over.

Oral antibiotics

These get prescribed for so many conditions now and often they are ineffective, but if you take the full dose like you are supposed to, you are going to kill off all the beneficial probiotic bacteria in your colon and then there is a good chance you will get a fungus infection (yeast) which can lead to severe problems. Anyway, make sure you replenish your probiotic bacteria if you take oral antibiotics. Kefir, acidophilus, fresh yogurt, raw sauerkraut. Do it. You don't want a fungus infection.

Raw or cooked?

In general, raw food is more nutritious. Most proteins, carbs, minerals, and fats seem to survive the cooking procedure, but vitamins can be destroyed by heat, also some enzymes. In the lab, we fed rats only on cooked food and they all died. Are there any advantages to cooking food? Light cooking or steaming does make some vegetables more easily digestible and loosens the fiber that binds up some of the nutrients. Some foods like grains and potatoes almost require cooking to be palatable.

Future of Food

Humans have to evolve away from meat eating. Way too inefficient a food source. I like growing kelp and other seaweeds in the sea. Big place. Let's use it to grow our food and stop domesticating the wild forests and prairies. Make the food from natural sources and make it so efficient. And every person on earth will be well-fed with good nutrition. Eat for health not pleasure.

Telomeres

This is a hot topic in health now. Telomeres are protective caps at the ends of each strand of DNA in every cell. The cells replenish themselves by dividing and each time they divide the telomere gets shorter. Finally, the cell can no longer divide and dies. It is called aging. Longer telomeres usually mean a longer life. The length is inherited from your parent's sperm and egg. They can also be shortened by stress, toxins, poor diet, obesity, and lack of exercise. Research is on now for a telomerase that can lengthen them, including possible natural sources. If you live long enough, they will have found a way to make you live longer.

Dementia linked to overprescribing drugs

A Harvard University report says "medications are common culprits in mental decline." As the body ages, the liver's efficiency when it comes to metabolizing drugs declines, and the kidneys do not eliminate them as quickly as they once did. This causes the drugs to accumulate in the body, which means those who take multiple medications are particularly susceptible to this effect. Included in the list of drugs that cause dementia-like symptoms are antidepressants, anti-anxiety medications, sedatives, corticosteroids, narcotics, antihistamines, cardiovascular drugs, and anticonvulsants.

Falling in love

When was the last time you fell in love? There is initially sort of a giddiness, flushed skin, racing heart, and sweaty palms. There are 3 chemicals released in the brain, dopamine, norepinephrine, and phenylethlamine. According to Helen Fisher of Rutgers U, the chemicals cause bliss, intense energy, sleeplessness, cravings, loss of appetite, and focused attention. What causes the release of this love cocktail? Through the optic nerve. Love is visual.

Repetitive intake

You should change and vary your habits of eating and drinking. Take a break and make a change. Even if it seems you are ingesting high quality food or juices, there may be something harmful in it. Maybe just a little bit, but if you do it every day, it could eventually cause you a problem. Don't do anything every day. Change your brands. Give your body a chance to replenish itself. What about repetitive stress? Not good. Repetitive movements? Dangerous. If you eat bread you should find two or more loaves that have good ingredients and fiber and alternate them. I don't like to eat the same bread every day.

Good bread

Had 3 responses to my facebook complaint that I cannot find any good bread and all three look very good. The first one I tried is from Good Harvest Bakery, 1500 Kossuth in Lafayette, In. Very good loaf, high fiber, no preservatives, no synthetics, no enriched anything. $5.85 per loaf. Long line of people buying the bread. Also serve breakfast and lunch at a few tables. Fresh ground 100% whole wheat flour, water, flax seed, millet, oat bran, sunflower seeds, wheat bran, yeast, sea salt Jenny and Jerry Lacy

Premature graying

If a person gets gray in their 20's or 30's, there is a good chance that they are deficient in PABA, Pantothenic acid, Biotin, Folic acid, or copper. The gray hair is a symptom and the deficiency can lead to something more destructive to the person unless corrected.

I have personally seen color restored by taking the supplements.

Farming in the sea

Bren Smith now operates one of the largest seaweed hatcheries in the country, with tanks full of developing kelp spores, and a processing room that comes alive in spring when he and his team bring in the harvest and get it ready for sale. Blanched in 170-degree water, kelp turns a vivid green and can then be sold fresh or frozen, sometimes in the form of noodles. Smith's customers include Google for their cafeteria, Yale University, and several restaurants and wholesalers. He has sold out the last four years.

Becoming a vegan

When I first stopped eating animal products, I went down to 135 pounds from 175. My ribs were sticking out and my chest looked emaciated. I talked to a vegetarian physician friend of mine and he examined me and said I seemed fine and that eventually my weight would return. And he was right. I gained my weight back and an extra 25 pounds that I am still trying to lose now. My body had to adjust to not eating meat. I fasted and cleansed myself and never went back.

Our normal flora

People think that, by washing, their skin is perfectly clean, but in actuality, our skins are completely covered by bacteria and some fungi and maybe other organisms, no matter how much you wash. If you scrubbed a small area with alcohol you would temporarily have a bare spot, but it would not take long for the flora to regrow over it. Sweat itself doesn't smell bad, but when the bacteria eat the sweat, their waste products can have a bad odor eventually. And we are also covered with microorganisms from our mouth to our anus. That is considered outside our body. Inside the body where the blood is should be sterile.

PABA

Para-aminobenzoic acid (PABA) can absorb ultraviolet (UV) light when applied to the skin and is used to treat abnormal heart rhythms, bacterial infection, seizures, nausea and vomiting, mental illnesses, stomach issues, and pain.

PABA is a potential treatment for the prevention of recurring cold sores. PABA may have blood-thinning, anti-inflammatory, anti-malarial, and anti-tumor effects, as well as potential coloring benefits for graying hair.

Prostate problems

The prostate gland manufactures many of the components of semen which are mixed with the sperm during ejaculation. If a man is not having orgasms, the fluid builds up in the prostate and can cause swelling and often impedes the passage of urine because the urethra goes right through the prostate. 85% of men experience prostate swelling when they get older and may require some kind of procedure to keep the urine flowing. In some cases, the swollen prostate can lead to cancer. It is best to keep it drained with some kind of regular sex

Sperm sample

If a man is to give a sperm sample in a scientific setting, how is it obtained? Some people think he is given his choice of some magazines and sent into a private room with a jar. No, that is not how it is done. The physician puts on a rubber glove and massages the man's prostate gland through the rectum and he will experience an ejaculation of his semen. He does not necessarily require an erection. The semen just sort of runs out while he is flaccid, but he does have a type of orgasm. The prostate is a secondary orgasmic center in men. This method provides scientific control of the collection and storage of the semen. A fertility clinic just doing a basic examination of the semen often uses the private room masturbatory collection method, but not a scientific facility.

Hypersexuality

Hypersexuality is a psychological condition. Maybe it is psycho-social. The root cause is not completely understood. Is it a defect or is it a gift? Does the condition need treatment? Does the afflicted person usually seek help? Or need help? Is there an imbalance in the person's brain chemistry? Certainly, it is not considered normal, but does that make it a pathology?

A salesperson assesses everyone as a potential source of income. That is considered normal and actually, a very socially desirable trait. The male satyr or female nymphomaniac sort of assesses everyone as a potential sexual partner. That is considered as a sickness and the person is usually avoided in a social situation.

Is the hypersexual individual born with that trait? Or did something happen to create the condition. Was there a trauma causing some kind of a breakout through the normal constraints? Or is it a spiritual situation that manifested physically as the person grew up. Were there indications in the person's childhood? Probably, yes.

Two identical twin boys crawling on the floor. One tries to look under the skirts of women in the room and one could care less. One gets erections when being bathed and one doesn't. One plays with girls as playmates and the other senses some kind of sexual attraction even at a very young age. Basically, they have the same genetic makeup. Why the difference in their interest in sexuality.

Is it an illness that needs treatment? No one knows. Just because one therapist says there needs treatment does not mean he is correct. If the hypersexual does not break any laws of the society, should they be subjected to corrective therapies? Should they be ostracized? Does a person have the right to live their life as they choose if they do nothing illegal, even though they probably are violating customs and moral codes that they might not see as applicable to their own needs.

It is a specialized condition. Maybe it is not an illness. Just a way that person lives their life. If they are not forceful or in violation of child sanctity, should they be classified and maybe punished in some way because they especially enjoy sex? They really can't help it. It is an integral part of their mental make-up. Sex addiction is sort of like a gambling addiction, but not quite, because there is another person involved, their sexual partner that may have thoughts that they have been violated, maybe because of the lack of emotional commitment.

Some people think there should be a punishment for everything, either by jurisprudence or by condemnation in the afterlife. Dante felt hypersexuals should be subjected to extreme sensuality in the afterlife because of their enjoyment of the gift of sexuality on earth.

Peanut butter

A woman I know had been feeding her kids garbage peanut butter like Jiff and Peter Pan and I pointed out the trashy ingredients because she had never bothered to read the labels. She bought some peanuts-only peanut butter and her 6 year old spit the first bite onto the floor and then the 4 year old did the same thing. They wanted the sugar.

Early Female Puberty

I have heard accounts of girls 9 years old starting their menstrual cycles. My generation they were like 12 or 13 and my mother's generation 14 or 15. What happened? I think it is the prevalence of using female hormones in the steers so the meat will be more tender. Many countries will not accept imports of American beef because of the hormones. And what about the boys who eat the beef? Well, I remember the WWII vets and they were tough guys. Most American guys are not like that nowadays. Just look at the entertainers and movie stars now and then.

Fast-Walk

Dr. Karl-Otto Aly, MD, took part in an experimental walk from Gothenburg to Stockholm in Sweden. The distance was 375 miles and it took him ten days of steady walking. What was unusual is that he fasted the entire time. No food whatsoever. Just water. The experiment was to determine the effects of fasting under conditions of severe stress. He felt stronger and had more vitality and vigor after the fast than before.

Mental health and raw foods

A research team in New Zealand found a significant association between consuming raw fruits and vegetables and better mental health outcomes. More raw food meant a better mood, life satisfaction and overall psychological well-being compared to eating cooked, canned or processed. Foods in their raw state deliver more micronutrients. Cooking fruits and vegetables can alter the bioavailability of nutrients which play an influential role in the neurotransmission systems involved in mood and well-being. Cooking and processing also diminish the quantity and activity of antioxidants. This too can negatively affect mental functioning.

Comfrey

When Germans immigrated here they brought seeds from their native country and one of the important ones was comfrey. They called it bone plant because it speeds the healing of bone problems like breaks when it is applied as a compress. I use it as a main ingredient in Dr. Cargill's European facial treatment because it contains allantoin which is found in the mother-to-be's amnionic fluid around her baby and it stimulates the growth of new tissue. And it does it to the skin of the face. It also is about the only plant that has Vitamin B 12 for blood manufacture. So drink some of the tea and hold it under the tongue.

Psoriasis

How about trying raw vegetables and fruits in season. Raw nuts and seeds, especially sesame seeds, pumpkin seeds, and sunflower seeds and cold-pressed oils from those seeds. Extra virgin olive oil. Drink the oils straight from a spoonful. No animal fats. No hydrogenated oils at all. Cranberry juice. Where possible apply sea water externally to the lesion. At least sea salt dissolved in water. Avoid frequent bathing and use no soap on the affected area. Salt bath with salt dissolved in the bath water. Lots of sunshine. External application of the seed oils. Juice fasting for at least a week.

One-a-day vitamins

These are the worst. Completely synthetic. Big molecules that probably will not be absorbed through the intestinal walls and end up in the toilet one way or another. Eat whole, natural vegetables and fruit and grains. Best to eat it raw if possible. Throw away those pills. The ONLY time you should take any kind of supplement is if you are showing sign of a deficiency in your diet. Then it has to be 100% natural and from a health food store, not a drug store.

Hypoglycemia

This is low blood sugar. Often physicians recommend high animal protein diet. It may help in controlling the condition, but will result in so many ill effects that you would be replacing one illness with others. Best to eat high natural plant carbohydrates. Eat 6-8 small meals per day. Fruit and vegetable juices should be diluted with 50% water. Avoid refined processed foods, especially table sugar.

Multiple Sclerosis

Hi Dr. Cargill: Do you have a diet plan for MS. I'm looking for best help for a best friend.

MS is a devastating disease that is probably auto-immune caused. The patient was exposed to an organism that has similar markers as their own cells that produce myelin, a covering around nerve fibers that sort of act like electrical insulation, so those nerve fibers begin to malfunction. At present there is no actual cure, but here are some dietary considerations:

fruits, berries, raw vegetables, especially beets, red cabbage, cucumbers, tomatoes, radishes, sauerkraut, sour pickles, any lactic acid veggies, cold-pressed seed oils, raw seeds, raw nuts, sprouts, and if he is not vegan, unsalted fresh butter, fertile eggs, raw goats milk, raw soured milk, homemade cottage cheese, liquid whey

No coffee, no chocolate, no salt, no spices, or no mustard, no pepper, no processed food, no sugar or any refined carbs. Try massage, hot baths and cold showers, swimming, mineral baths, maybe steam or sauna.

Itchy skin

Dry skin. If you don't see a crop of bright, red in the itchy area, dry skin is a likely cause. Dry skin usually results from older age or environmental factors such as long-term use of air conditioning or central heating, and washing or bathing too much.

Skin conditions and rashes. Many skin conditions itch, including eczema (dermatitis), psoriasis, scabies, lice, chickenpox and hives. The itching usually affects specific areas and is accompanied by other signs, such as red, irritated skin or bumps and blisters.

Internal diseases. Itchy skin can be a symptom of an underlying illness. These include liver disease, kidney failure, iron deficiency anemia, thyroid problems and cancers, including leukemia and lymphoma. The itching usually affects the whole body. The skin may look otherwise normal except for the repeatedly scratched areas.

Nerve disorders. Conditions that affect the nervous system — such as multiple sclerosis, diabetes mellitus, pinched nerves and shingles (herpes zoster) — can cause itching.

Irritation and allergic reactions. Wool, chemicals, soaps and other substances can irritate the skin and cause itching. Sometimes the substance, such as poison ivy or cosmetics, causes an allergic reaction. Food allergies also may cause skin to itch.

Drugs. Reactions to drugs, such as antibiotics, antifungal drugs or narcotic pain medications, can cause widespread rashes and itching.

Pregnancy. During pregnancy, some women experience itchy skin, especially on the abdomen and thighs. Also, itchy skin conditions, such as dermatitis, can worsen during pregnancy.

Excessive Sleeping

There is not a lot of really scientific material available on this subject. There is not even a consistent definition as to what is excessive. So it is hard to make any kind of judgements. I had an associate who seemed healthy and alert, but claimed to require 12 hours of sleep every day in order to function. If she had a reason to necessarily get 6 or 8 hours of sleep, then she would get up, but would make up for it the next day. She loved to sleep and she had an old dog that matched her hour for hour. I do know that carbon dioxide slowly builds up in the blood when we are sleeping so once we are past 8 hours of sleeping, it becomes more difficult to wake up. If a person sleeps more than 16 hours, the carbon dioxide levels will be so high that they will never just awaken by themselves and they will actually sleep to death. What is normal? All experiments I have read claim that the normal sleeping cycle for humans is 8 hours.

Potato Chips

Why I don't eat potato chips. I used to live in far northwest Minnesota in the potato country. None of the farmers eat the potatoes that they grow for the chipper factory. I used to eat them because my girlfriend worked on a potato harvester and brought some home every night. When we boiled them they gave off a green foam, but we still used them to make lefse which I loved. The potato farmers all buy *organically grown potatoes for their families.*

BPA

The container soda typically comes in is deeply problematic. Nearly all cans used by the U.S. beverage industry contain bisphenol A, commonly known as BPA. Here's how *Scientific American* describes it: "In recent years dozens of scientists around the globe have linked BPA to myriad health effects in rodents: mammary and prostate cancer, genital defects in males, early onset of puberty in females, obesity, and even behavior problems such as attention-deficit hyperactivity disorder." The Canadian government recently declared BPA toxic. BPA is associated with "decreased sexual desire [among men], more difficulty having an erection, lower ejaculation strength and lower level of overall satisfaction with sex life.

Gall bladder cleanse

This is a true story of one of my patients. His mother had recently died from complications of a surgery t remove gall stones from her gall bladder. Now my patient himself was diagnosed with gall stones blocking the release of bile from his gall bladder. Bile is released when we ingest fats. I suggested to him that he drink only apple cider for a week and then on the 7th day drink an entire bottle of extra virgin olive oil. Since he ate no fat for the week, the bile built up a large supply in the gall bladder and when he drank all that oil the bile and the gall stones came rushing out into his intestines and right into the toilet. He gathered up the little green stones and showed me. I was amazed at how many stones and the size of them. He has had no problem since.

Acne

Pores become clogged with sebum oil and dirt. The sebum has a lot of oleic acid which is similar to that found in olive oil. Clean it with an oil high in linoleic acid : safflower, black cumin, hemp seed, pumpkin seed, rose hip oil, soybean oil, wheat germ oil and add some of it to your diet.

Dr. Cargill's Holistic Secrets to Bountiful Good Health

There seems to be 3 indisputable factors in achieving a state of good health. Diet, exercise, and rest. You don't need flu vaccinations to avoid getting sick. You just need a strong immune system. A way to fight off germs that you are exposed to. It can be done by anyone, and does not take much effort. Developing good health actually can be very enjoyable.

Probably the most important factor is your nutritional intake. Do you need meat? No. In fact, it seems that people who eat meat are sick more often than plant-only eaters.

Eat for Health

It is like where do you place your values. What is most important to you? Making as much money as possible? Admiration? Sexual love? Wisdom? Possessions? Posterity? Happiness? How about your health? Don't you really feel that enjoyment of any of those other goals is dependent upon being in a state of good health? What good is gold if you feel miserable?

It all comes down to what you eat. There are other factors, of course, like the air you breathe and the water you drink, that may have a big effect on your health. And how about your mental attitude towards things?

www.ingramcontent.com/pod-product-compliance
Lightning Source LLC
Chambersburg PA
CBHW031052250726
48655CB00004B/1397